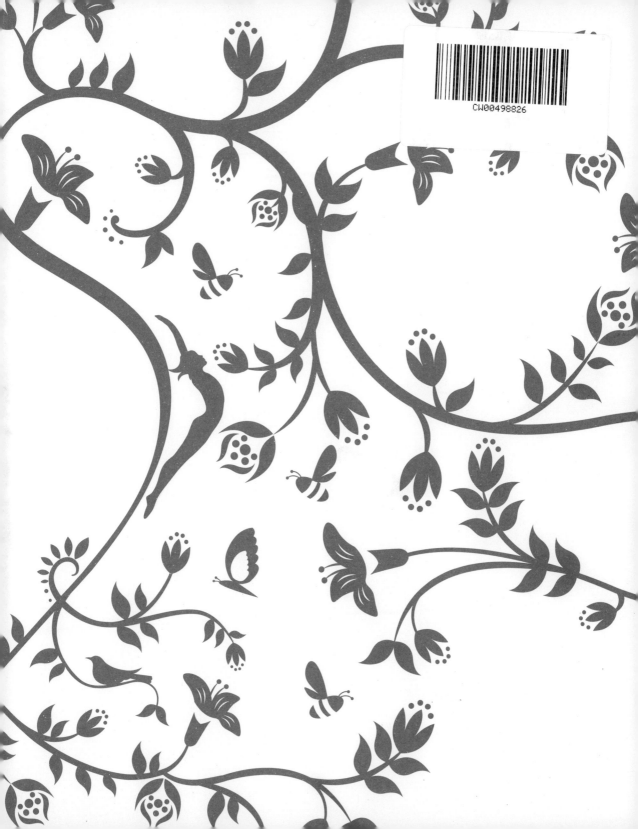

Cleanse Nurture Restore

with Herbal Tea

Frances Lincoln Limited
A subsidiary of Quarto Publishing Group UK
74–77 White Lion Street
London N1 9PF

Cleanse, Nurture, Restore with Herbal Tea
© Frances Lincoln Limited 2016
Text © Sebastian Pole 2016
Photographs © Kim Lightbody 2016
Commissioning editor: Zena Alkayat

First Frances Lincoln edition 2016

A catalogue record for this book is available
from the British Library.

ISBN 978-0-7112-3829-9

Printed and bound in China

1 2 3 4 5 6 7 8 9

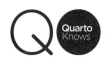

FRANCES
LINCOLN

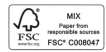

Quarto is the authority on a wide range of topics.

Quarto educates, entertains and enriches the lives of
our readers – enthusiasts and lovers of hands-on living.

www.QuartoKnows.com

Cleanse Nurture Restore

with Herbal Tea

Sebastian Pole

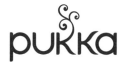

Contents

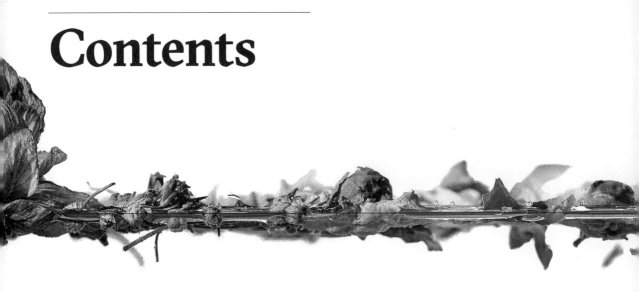

07
Introduction

11
The language of herbs

15
The doctrine of signatures

19
The perfect blend

23
The art of making herbal tea

27
Helpful herbal terms

28
Ailments & Elixirs

30
Cleanse & Detox

48
Nourish & Digest

66
Energise & Rejuvenate

90
Peace & Harmony

110
Joy & Happiness

132
Defend & Protect

158
Man, Woman & Child

184
Beyond Tea

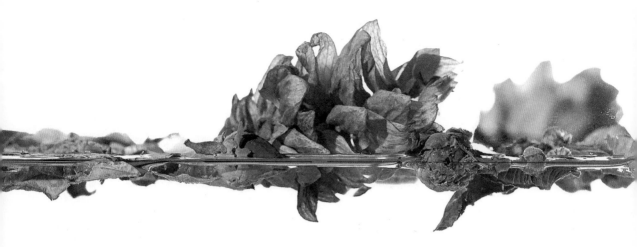

211
About Ayurveda

222
Pukkapedia

231
Where do herbs come from?

232
Suppliers & Practitioners

234
Index

240
Thank yous

Disclaimer

The author and publisher disclaim any liability arising from the use or misuse of the information contained in this book. The book is not to be relied on for diagnosis or treatment of any disease. It also should not be relied on for medical or other healthcare advice and has been compiled by way of general guidance in relation to the specific subjects addressed. The reader should seek professional advice from a qualified herbalist or experienced medical doctor on the specific subjects addressed, as well as information on up-to-date practice, laws and regulations. In addition, anyone who is pregnant or trying to conceive should seek professional advice prior to using these recipes.

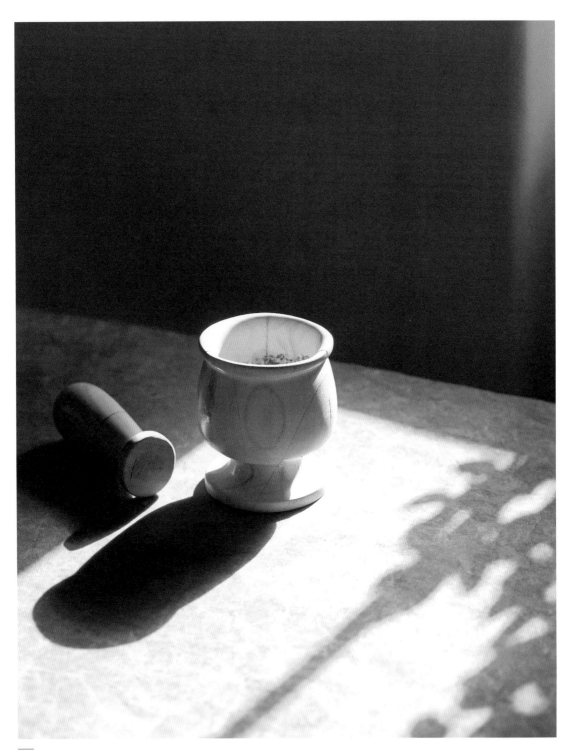

Introduction

Welcome to *Cleanse, Nurture, Restore with Herbal Tea* – it's filled with tempting recipes brimming with nature's healing powers. Beautiful to look at, easy to make and delicious to drink, each herbal tea infusion harnesses the health-giving brilliance of our botanical kingdom. So if you want to learn how to improve your life with a few simple herbal blends, then you are holding the right book. In it, I will take you on a gentle stroll through the world of herbs, teaching you how to mix some herbal classics, as well as feed your budding enthusiasm with more creative combinations.

I first experienced the power of plants when I was eighteen. I had been travelling in India and had a terrible bout of 'Delhi belly'. An Ayurvedic doctor gave me a simple powder of licorice root, shatavari root and amla fruit to take. It cleared me up in a few days and I immediately wanted to find out how the blend had worked. Ever since then I have spent my life dedicated to learning about herbs as well as sharing my knowledge and inspiration. Supporting thousands of patients in my clinic (and having served hundreds of millions of cups of Pukka tea), I am left with an overwhelming feeling of gratitude for how much joy and sustenance herbs bring to people.

Plants have been at the centre of human health forever and it feels like we are only just rediscovering how important they are to living well today. Helping to nourish, cleanse, rejuvenate and restore your whole system, herbs can be used for both optimising your health as well as getting you better if you are unwell: in other words, they can be food as well as medicine. Their life-enhancing properties are simple to bring into your everyday life, and one of my favourite ways to do this is by making herbal blends and drinking their delicious infusions.

The history of medicine is largely the history of herbal medicine. If human life were a 24-hour clock, then herbs have been at the heart of all health traditions for 23 hours 59 minutes. Imagine journeying back 10,000 years: we would be living at the mercy of nature, and the care and protection of our loved ones would be high up our to-do list. We would be dependent on the shamans, healers and wisewomen for talismans and incantations as well as herbal brews and poultices to help heal all manner of ills. And we would have to understand the natural world around us so that we could stay healthy. Out of the ancient intuitive folklore tradition grew the great cultures of medicine from Asia, Europe and the Americas collated by such famous doctors as Hippocrates, Galen, Culpeper, Charaka, Sushruta, Huang Di and Li Shizhen in Greek, European, Chinese and Ayurvedic medicine. These giants of natural healing harnessed the folklore insights into codified and systematic scientific medical traditions. Many elements of these traditions are so profound that, having engaged in the longest and most successful human clinical trial in history, they are still practised by herbalists today. This book will show you how this theory can work in practice.

Ever since I started Pukka Herbs in 2001 with my Pukka partner Tim Westwell, we have been overwhelmed by positive feedback: people love drinking our teas. It's amazing to be able to spend your time doing what you love, but it's even more special when others love it too. Our goal is to continue to serve the best cup of herbal tea we can by bringing you some of the world's finest herbs. We've wanted these teas to be as good as the cups of tea we serve to our friends and family – in fact, many of the Pukka teas have been directly inspired by the blends initially created for our loved ones.

I have had the privilege of blending all the Pukka teas myself and each one has a story: some have been influenced by my work in my herbal clinic, some are traditional classics, some are just for pleasure. Making these teas for you to enjoy is one of the most important things I do, and as with anything you want to do well, there is a lot to consider: how to consistently grow supreme quality herbs while considering long-term sustainability in every herb; how to make it taste exceptional; how to bring the best health benefit; and how to create a feeling of contentment in every cup.

I have visited hundreds of organic farms over the years and witnessed again and again how farming organically can bring immeasurable benefit to people, plants and planet. I have travelled far and wide to find herbs that are the best they can be. And in among the hullabaloo and chaos of life I have felt inspired and

encouraged by some incredible farms, enthusiastic farmers and remarkable herbs.

Back in my herbal clinic, these plants transform people's lives by bringing them greater vitality and peace. I have seen the breathless breathe, the sleepless sleep and the exhausted become reenergised. These transformations are testament to the intelligence within plants and show us that traditional medicine can really help us balance our health and support us as we journey through life. My overarching experience of using herbs myself is that they help me to be a better person: more aware, more present, more engaged. Because herbs help to remove imbalance and pain they essentially bring more happiness into the world, and I'll always drink another cup of happiness.

This is really a book to enjoy. There are dozens of herbs to discover, the language of nature to learn and a whole lot of satisfaction to experience. It's also a book to take seriously, as you need to make sure you use the herbs appropriately. This means following the guidelines in the book as well as using your instinct. Herbs are powerful ingredients that can change how you feel. You will get the most from them if you use your inner wisdom as well as your common sense. When you first plan on making a tea, consider whether the measure of each herb suggested is suitable for you. For example, the spices are hot, so depending on your taste for a fiery sensation, you may wish to adjust the amount. And be aware of the cleansing herbs – these will send you to the loo, so make sure you are ready for that. I have explained the effects of the herbs in each recipe, but do remember that you are unique so it's best to use your own judgement. The recipes are for you to use as a base to build on as your confidence grows so tweak or adjust them in line with your tastes and needs.

These initial pages introduce the world of herbs and help you to understand their myriad benefits. They also cover the art of creating a perfect herbal tea blend, a glossary of useful terms used throughout the book and advice on dosages and how to make the recipes. At the back of the book (from p211) I've included an overview of Ayurveda and some Ayurvedic inspiration. You can read these sections in their entirety, dip into them at your leisure or refer back to them when you have a question or want to find out a little bit more about the principles that go into making a great cup of herbal tea.

The rest of the book is split into chapters that cover the different functions and aims of the teas. Using traditional herbal medicine and some of the principles of Ayurveda, I have included recipes for making herbal teas for just about every need, from improving your digestion and helping you sleep, to reawakening your mojo. Think of each recipe as an idea that you can adjust depending on your tastes or requirements (be it for the pleasure of the flavour or to address an ailment). All you need to do is buy, grow or forage some of the herbs, weigh them out like any

recipe, put them in a teapot, add some hot water and relax while the magic happens. As the herbs brew, their colourful pigments, aromatic essential oils and other powerful ingredients will seep into the hot water and create something very special: an infusion of botanical delight; a cup of incredible herbal tea.

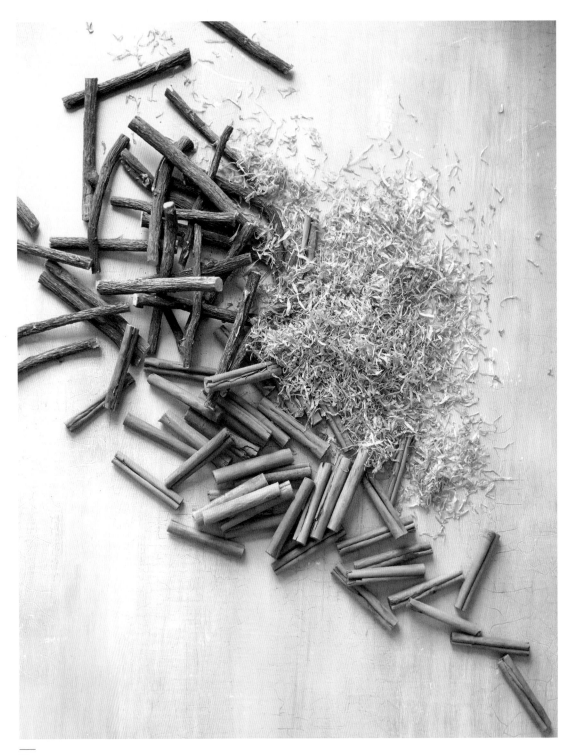

The language of herbs

The world of herbs is as broad as it is deep. Herbalism is an integral part of our evolution and is effectively the history of human medicine. So if you want to understand the herbal tea recipes on a level that's deeper than just 'ingredients and water', learning about the language of herbs should give you some fascinating insights.

One of herbalism's enduring attributes is how simple it is to understand. Being based on natural designs, all of the language, systems and principles of herbal medicine are second nature to us. Or they would be had we grown up living close to nature… In the absence of firsthand experience, a little theory will aid your practice. So before we delve into the recipes, it's useful to cover the basics and building blocks in order for you to learn the language of herbs and how they can help us.

If you want to get a specific result you need to know what plant, or combination of plants, will lead to success in any given situation, as well as how and why they might work. A useful way to understand how plants work is to think about them from three different perspectives. The first is the natural view: that 'they just work' because they have evolved to help themselves as well as us. The second is the phytochemical view: that plants' chemical compounds initiate a healing response in us. And the third is the energetic view: that plants have recognisable properties and characteristics that have an effect on our bodies. These three approaches require completely different ways of thinking about plants, but each can contribute to a deeper appreciation of how they work.

The natural way

The natural view is that herbs are good for us because they are good for themselves. Imagine you are a plant, rooted in one spot and unable to move when faced with marauding animals, adverse weather and invading microbes. You would work out pretty quickly how to defend yourself, or you would die. And the plants have done just that. Ever since the earliest blue-green algae/cyanobacteria (such as spirulina) channelled the sun's energy 2 billion years ago, green plants have been harnessing the energy of life. They have used this energy to flourish into mosses, ferns, fungi and – a few hundred million years later – hundreds of thousands of flowering species all with self-protective abilities. Just as the resin that exudes from a damaged tree trunk can stop infection from damaging the tree, so many tree resins can heal our wounds and ward off infections. It's for this reason that myrrh (a tree resin) was considered to be the most important antibiotic in the ancient world – Jesus wasn't just given any old gifts.

As animals evolved together with the plant kingdom they learned how to use each other for mutual advantage. For example, it's testimony to the success of this evolutionary relationship that plants have always appreciated animals' seed-spreading skills, while animal and human bodies are able to benefit from a plant's natural healing qualities. Primates and other animals use various species of herbs for specific health needs: they know herbs for an upset tummy, herbs for wounds, herbs for pregnancy. As we learned to tap into nature's innate properties, we also learned one of the great secrets of life: that plants help our body and mind to heal. Our relationship with plants is so successful that the health of our cardiovascular, digestive, immune, respiratory, nervous, endocrine and psychological systems is largely dependent on plants. How we think, feel, procreate and heal are all influenced by the herbs and plants we eat and drink. Herbs just work, naturally.

The phytochemical way

Plants have developed both procreative and protective compounds – phytochemicals – that help them create future generations as well as protect them against damage from a plethora of microbes. For example, our good friend peppermint has evolved powerful essential oils to ward off fungal invasions, while ashwagandha root produces steroid-like compounds that build fertility, helping it to spread its seed. The great variety of phytochemicals found in medicinal plants are made from only a few chemical elements. The major ones are carbon, hydrogen and oxygen, others include nitrogen or sulfur, and occasionally metal ions (e.g. magnesium, calcium or phosphorus).

The key thing to understand, though, is that plants create a host of natural chemical compounds that have an effect on the human body and are classed as secondary metabolites. Examples include caffeine, essential oils, antioxidants and steroids. These natural compounds are not the primary carbohydrate, protein or fat that our body needs, but other not-essential-to-life but still-very-important-to-life molecular structures. One way to think of molecular structures is as patterns of energy in a relationship. These patterns of energy carry information from the plant to our human receptors and physiological systems.

Because of the millions of years of evolutionary history between humans and plants, we can benefit from a plant's phytochemicals too. And phytochemicals are proven to work as they form the basis for hundreds of drugs. Some well-known examples include morphine from opium and taxol from the yew tree.

Amazingly, some herbs have 1,000-plus phytochemical compounds found at very low levels of concentration. And given our 10 million-year human evolution, it's no surprise that we respond very well to a wide range of low-dose phytochemicals. If there are 1,000 compounds in a plant and we once ate a diet of around 150 species of plants (compared with around 20 today), we are familiar with around 150,000 plant compounds. In contrast, modern medicine has no precedent in our evolutionary history, and while a high dose of a pharmaceutical drug may be valuable in an emergency, herbs are the medicines we evolved to use for our everyday health.

The energetic way

Plant species have a character unique to themselves that, rather like someone you know well, has a recognisable personality. Some are energising, some are calming some are restorative. This understanding of how plants behave is called 'herbal energetics' and relates to our experience of how the plant affects us: does it heat us up or cool a fever? Does it moisten our skin or dry up a runny nose? Does it rejuvenate us or weigh us down and help us to sleep? Herbal energetics is about how the herb makes us feel.

To discover how it will make us feel, we don't just need to know what is in it, we need to know 'who it is'. And to find this out, like a good scientist, we have to observe and learn what the plant does. Experiment for yourself and see: some plants are lively (chew some ginger), and some are much more mellow (try sipping some chamomile tea). Some awaken our hearts (like a beautiful rose), and others make us happy (too many to mention, but lemon balm and tulsi can make you sing from the treetops).

Traditional health systems (such as Ayurveda) teach us to open our senses and read the language of nature. They offer insights into how we can read plants and how we can benefit from them. For example, finding out how plants cope with extreme conditions can reveal a lot about their beneficial health properties. Ginseng can survive through the harshest winters – and it can also warm us up. Aloe vera thrives in the hot desert – and it can soothe our burns. Cinnamon is happy in the humid jungle – and its drying heat can help protect us from damp and cold weather by increasing circulation in our bodies. Sweet elderberries thrive in damp forests – and they help to keep us healthy through the winter by clearing mucus from our chest and protecting us from viruses (it actually protects us from over 11 types of flu virus).

It's worth remembering that ultimately plants share life with us and we have developed complex physiological and psychological systems to understand them. We just need to open our hearts and minds as we see, smell, taste, touch and listen to life.

So as you go on to make these teas and explore herbalism, take a little time to notice how plants affect you, and a whole new world will open up. Some call this new world 'the life force' – one that carries the innate healing power of nature. In Ayurveda it's called *prana*, in China it's *qi* and in the European tradition it's known as *vis medicatrix naturae* (the healing power of nature). In Japan, the concept of *shinrin-yoku* (which translates as 'taking in the forest air' or 'forest bathing') suggests that being in nature can improve your health. There is a whole new language in herbalism – and it's one you already largely know.

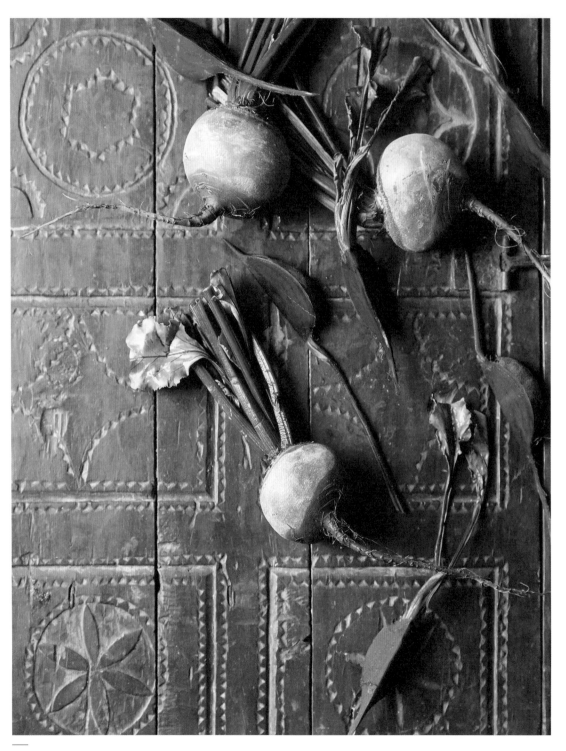

The doctrine of signatures is an idea beloved by some herbalists. It developed in traditional folk medicine when people believed the 'creator' had laid out signs so that we could read nature and understand what effect plants have on us.

The doctrine of signatures

According to the doctrine of signatures, with careful observation you can learn the uses of a plant from some aspect of its shape, colour or natural habitat. Some herbalists love this idea as, whether it's true or not (not *all* the principles hold true *all* of the time), it can help you remember what certain herbs do. There are many examples of this, so below I've mentioned a few of my favourites.

Learning from the shape
- Walnuts resemble a human brain and are excellent for promoting healthy brain function (they are packed with brain-friendly omega-3 fatty acids).
- Garlic has hollow stems and is good for respiratory disorders (it has potent antimicrobial properties).
- Fresh ginger root echoes the shape of a stomach and is one of nature's greatest digestive tonics, helping the assimilation of nutrients, removal of pathogens (microorganisims that cause bacteria and viruses) and fighting against nausea.
- Gotu kola leaf looks like a cross-section of the brain and has a long history of use for improving memory. Phytochemists have now shown it can enhance cognitive function.

- St John's wort leaf has lots of pore-like perforation on its leaves, making it useful for 'holes' in the skin such as cuts or bruises. It's also good at letting the light in and banishing the blues.

Learning from the colour
- Plants with yellow flowers or roots, such as dandelion flower or turmeric root, were traditionally believed to be good for the liver and to cure 'yellow' conditions, such as jaundice.
- Red plants, such as hawthorn berry or beetroot, were traditionally used for heart and blood disorders. Both hawthorn berry and beetroot are now acknowledged as cardiac tonics that strengthen blood flow and heart muscle strength.
- Plants with creamy-white coloured flowers, such as elderflower and yarrow, are considered to be good for expelling 'creamy' mucus and discharges from the body.

Learning from the habitat
Where a plant grows can sometimes give you insights into how it can help you. Take willow for example: it thrives in damp waterlogged meadows

and is good for arthritis, a painful disease often involving swelling of the joints that is exacerbated by damp weather. Herbs like aloe vera and shatavari root grow in a dry climate and can help to moisten dryness anywhere in the body, while herbs growing in a wet climate like elecampane root and willow bark can help to dry damp-wetness, like when we have a cough or arthritic swelling. Herbs growing in a cold climate (like ginseng and horseradish) can help warm us up, while herbs growing in a hot climate (like neem and andrographis) help cool us down. There are quite a few exceptions to this rule, which is why the doctrine of signatures is just a mysterious and poetic idea to help us connect with a plant's character and to remind us what it does.

Learning from the name

As well as the doctrine of signatures, you can have fun picking apart the names of herbs. Prior to the advent of Linnaeus's formal botanical classifications, herbs were known by many different names according to identifiable factors including taste, smell, shape, the specific part of a plant, habitat, history or animal part (such as lion's tooth – now known as dandelion). Whether it's an old folklore name, Sanskrit or Latin, there will probably be a clue telling you what the herb does, or what it tastes or smells like. It's a simple reminder that the senses were paramount in developing traditional herbal healing. Here are a few of the best examples.

Taste Licorice is the root of the plant named *Glycyrrhiza glabra* in Latin and *yashtimadhu* in Sanskrit. Both mean 'sweet root' or 'sweet stick', which reflects its sweet flavour. Andrographis's traditional names are *mahatikta* or 'king of bitters', referring to its extremely bitter taste.

Smell Ashwagandha means 'smelling like a horse' in Sanskrit – which it does – but its name also refers to the belief that it will make you strong like a horse.

Shape The nutritious micro-algae spirulina is named after its spiral-shaped swirls.

Colour Another name for tulsi (holy basil) is *krishna*, meaning 'black' – this reflects the dark colour of its leaves and stems. The nutritional algae chlorella's name appropriately means 'little green'.

Effect The botanical name for chamomile is *Matricaria recutita*. *Matrix* is Latin for 'womb', nodding to chamomile's ability to aid gynaecological complaints. The bark of the guelder rose (*Viburnum opulus*) has long been used to treat menstrual cramps and goes by the common name cramp bark. Motherwort (*Leonarus cardiaca*) is thought to be beneficial for mothers pre- and post-labour. And the Latin indication for the species, *Cardiaca*, suggests it is good for the heart (palpitations from anxiety). The Latin for ginseng is *Panax ginseng*, referring to it being a cure-all 'panacea'.

The doctrine of signatures

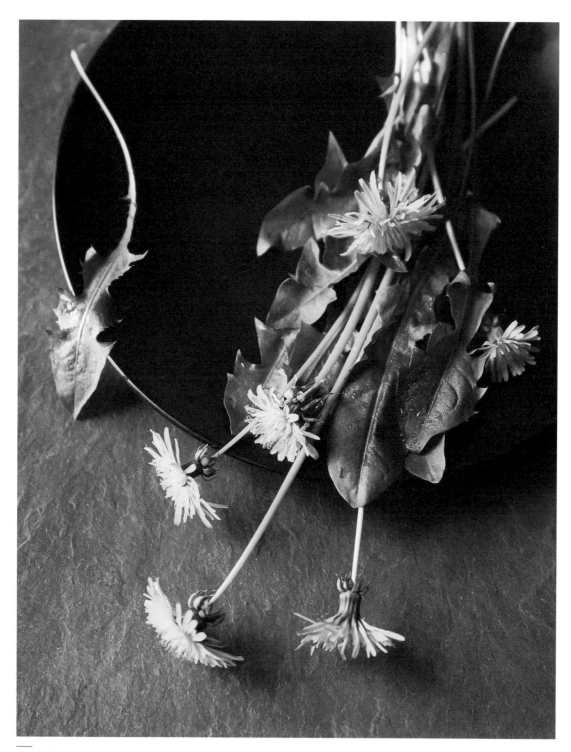

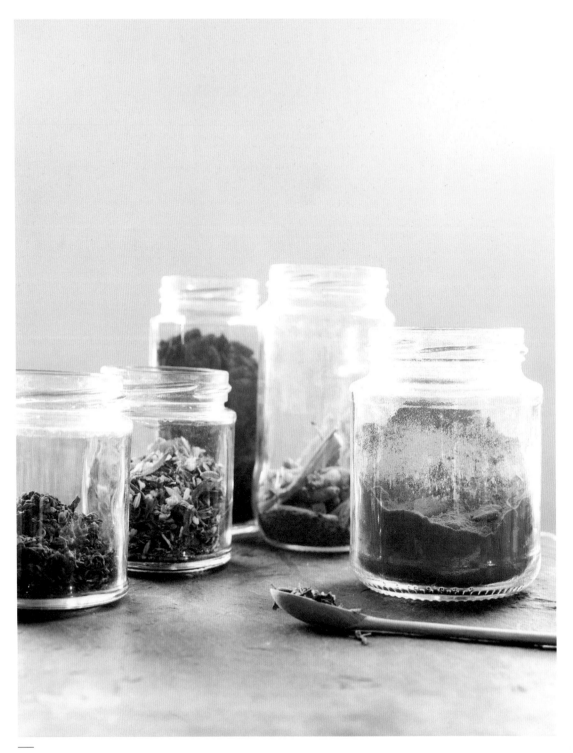

Herbalists often use herbs in combination to create a blend or a formula – or you could think of them as 'concoctions' or 'potions' to summon up thoughts of a powerful antidote. These blends are based on the idea that there is strength in numbers and that diversity can help us be safer as well as stronger.

The perfect blend

There is power in working together and it's a firm belief that the whole is greater than the sum of its parts, or as I like to say: 1 + 1 = 3 where two herbs used together gives you the power of three. The use of herbal blends is fundamental to the philosophy as well as the success of Western herbalism, traditional Chinese medicine and Ayurveda. Synergy is assumed to play a part in the benefits of all herbal treatments.

A synergistic effect can be between multiple herbs that have different functions, or indeed the same function – for example, it has been shown that ginseng root and ginkgo leaf (both used to aid cognitive function) have a more potent effect when used together than when used alone.

But synergy isn't exclusive to different herbs working together. Scientists have also proven what the ancient masters knew through instinct and experimentation: synergy also takes place between the constituents within a single herb, enhancing some aspects and limiting extremes in others. For example, dandelion leaf is a strong diuretic but is also high in potassium (which helps maintain cellular fluid balance). So unlike pharmaceutical diuretics, dandelion leaf does not lead to electrolyte imbalance.

The yoga of tea
The yoga of tea is all about the perfect cup of tea. This will probably be different for all of us, but for me the perfect cup of tea needs to tick three boxes: it has to serve a purpose, it has to be of exceptional quality and it has to benefit people, plants and planet.

Serving a purpose is all about the *intention* of the tea. Do you want something calming? A pick-me-up? Or a digestif? Whenever I make a new herbal tea, I always spend time contemplating which herbs can be combined to best serve a purpose.

Exceptional quality is all about the plant: how has it been grown? Has it been covered in pesticides? Or is it organic? Is it a medicinal grade herb? Or, like most herbal teas, just bog-standard food grade? Has it been tested for levels of active essential oils and colourful pigments? For me, the answer is that it has to be organic (that is the best and most sustainable system of farming in the world today). And at Pukka we grow a grade of herbs that is called a 'pharmacopoeial medicinal grade' – this technical term means that the herb meets high standards for quality and consistently tastes great.

And finally the benefit of the tea relates to whether the tea is doing good – to me, to the farmer who grew the herbs and to the planet. If I know that these touchstones are reached, I am one happy herbsmith.

A balanced recipe

Making a tempting tea that is good for you is a bit like cooking a healthy meal: you need to combine a range of textures, tastes and experiences to create something that is nourishing and delicious. It helps to have a clear idea of what purpose the tea will serve and who you want to benefit from drinking it. I always take time to reflect on this before I start blending. If what you want to achieve is simply a tasty tea, it should be fairly easy to concoct. For more serious situations, you could write down ideas or spend time meditating on the solution.

The pattern I was taught to help formulate a blend takes in some wonderful characters. There's a King, a Prince, a Harmoniser, a Digester and a Messenger.

Start by selecting the lead herb or herbs that will act like the King and essentially be at the forefront of the tea. These herbs should be delivering the strongest and most specific effect. The King should be the main herb by weight and by effect.

Back this selection up with a supporting herb that behaves like a helpful Prince. These herbs will work in a synergistic way to enhance the power of the King. They should have specific aims, but be at a lower dose to the King herbs. Herbs like chamomile flowers, cinnamon bark or nettle leaf are often Kings and Princes.

Next you need to bring in a Harmoniser. A harmonising herb helps balance any extremes among the King and Prince herbs. It can reduce any extreme

flavours or effects – for example, if the lead herbs are a bit 'heating' or 'intense', then a harmoniser like sweet licorice can ameliorate such effects or flavours.

To help all of these herbs be assimilated into the body, you need to add a Digester. Digester herbs might include fennel seed or ginger root.

And finally, to send this formula somewhere specific in your body, add in a Messenger. Some herbs go directly to some organs and tissues – for example, some are specific for digestion (like ginger), some for the lungs (like thyme), some for the nervous system (like lemon balm). Add these as appropriate.

As an example, I've broken down the Digestive Detox With A Twist recipe on p39 below. And it's worth noting that most of the recipes in the book follow this structure.

KING: Aniseed 4g
KING: Fennel seed 4g
PRINCE: Cardamom pod 3g
PRINCE: Dandelion root 2g
HARMONISER: Licorice root 1g
DIGESTER: Celery seed 1g
MESSENGER: Lemon juice a twist

Use these ideas as just that: ideas. It may seem daunting to create your own blends, but by learning the basic language of herbs and getting to know how the herbs work, you will develop instincts. Over time, your intuition will grow in confidence and you can take the basic principles you've learned and combine them with firsthand expertise to create truly tailor-made recipes.

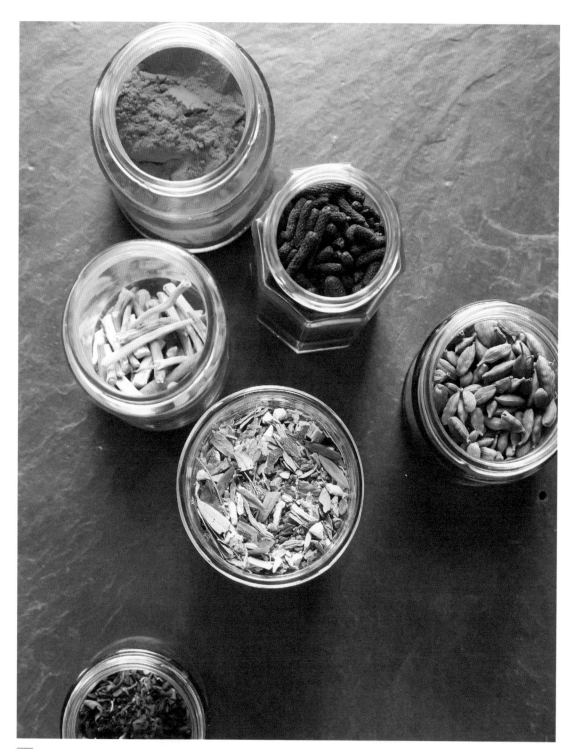

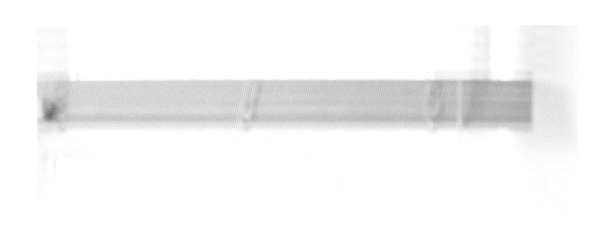

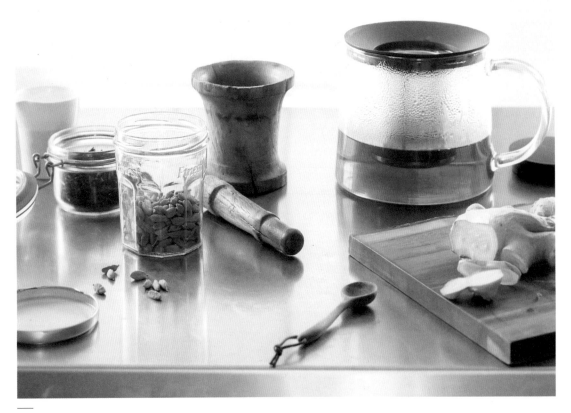

Just as selecting incredible organic herbs is important for a great cup of tea, so are the minute details of preparation, such as the amount of herbs in each cup, the shape and size of the herbs, the infusion time, the quality of water, the water temperature, the teapot... the company.

The art of making herbal tea

Ingredients

All of the herbs listed in the recipes are dried unless otherwise stated. The roots (ginger, turmeric, licorice) should all be used in their ground form unless otherwise stated. Sometimes fresh herbs are best – these have clearly been indicated with 'fresh' – so use them if you can get them. If you can't, just use dried herbs. While the ingredients are not the only part of a delicious and healthy cup of tea, they are the most important part. The tea will only be as good as the ingredients you put in it. Organic herbs are more potent than herbs grown with artificial fertilisers and pesticides, so make sure they are organic. You also want them to be brimming with goodness, so the herbs you use should look vibrant and smell bright and as they should.

Water and how to boil it

Water should be fresh, pure, clear, odourless and low in minerals, so it's best to use a water filter before making your tea. Getting a temperature-controlled kettle is a good way of ensuring you don't waste energy while you boil water for your cuppa.

Really hot water extracts more bitter and astringent compounds, making the tea (especially green tea) taste harsh, while water that is too cool is lacking the power to entice the flavours out of the herbs, making the tea taste weak. Overboiling your water causes the minerals to escape the solution and collect as a film on the surface. Overheating can upset the balance between the stronger tannins and some of the subtle volatile oils and amino acids in the herbs. More importantly, overboiling lowers the oxygen content in the water, which reduces its ability to convert the delicate aromatic compounds into tasty experiences.

Herbal teas should be made with freshly boiled water at a temperature of around 90–95°C / 195–205°F. More delicate herbs like lemon balm and lemon verbena can be infused at slightly lower temperatures; harder woody barks like licorice and cinnamon at slightly higher temperatures. When making delicate teas such as chamomile, mint or green teas, you should use freshly boiled water that has been left to cool a bit.

- Green tea 80–85°C / 175–185°F
- Oolongs around 85–90°C / 185–195°F
- Black teas around 95°C / 205°F

Infusion times

- Delicate aromatic flowers, leaves and seeds need less infusion time: 5–10 minutes
- Harder fruits, roots and barks need longer infusion times: 10–20 minutes

Shape and size

- Finely cut herbs infuse more quickly, large-cut herbs more slowly
- Hard herbs, like roots and barks, need to be finely cut if you want to infuse them in water. They can also be decocted (i.e. simmered or heated to extract their goodness). Keep a lid on the pan to avoid too much water and goodness escaping.
- Soft herbs should be infused. They too can be decocted, but only for short periods of time because otherwise they will lose their flavour.

Weighing

The measures of herbs in the recipes are listed in small quantities. For accuracy you need digital scales. I've listed them in metric measures (grams), but you can also use a teaspoon (particularly if you're more familiar with imperial measures in ounces). Once you have a bit more experience you can use the 'pinch' method and estimate in very general weights, and follow up by measuring. Using a teaspoon and pinch method will depend on the plant part, how finely it's been cut and your hand or spoon size. See the chart below for the closest conversion.

Dosages and quantities

How much you should have of what herb or tea and when you should have it are key questions when it comes to making and drinking herbal teas. While there

Gram to teaspoon conversion				
Plant form	1 teaspoon (5ml)	½ teaspoon (2.5ml)	1 pinch	1 handful
Powder	3.5g	1.75g	2g	Not recommended!
Root	3g	1.5g	5g	15g
Bark	2g	1g	4g	15g
Leaf	1g	0.5g	3g	10g
Flower	1g	0.5g	3g	10g
Fruit	1.5g	0.75g	1.5g	12g
Seed	2.5g	1.25g	2.5g	12g

The art of making herbal tea

are some minimum amounts needed to get a suitable flavour and effect from a herb, there are also maximum recommended amounts for some herbs so they are not too strong. Please see the specific information on each herb (note especially senna, cinnamon, licorice). But you won't go too far wrong if you follow this rule:

- As a daily drink: 1–5g of a herb, consumed 3 times per day
- For stronger therapeutic benefits: 5–10g of a herb, consumed 3 times per day

Determining dosages for children

There are some specific rules for determining dosages for children. Age is one consideration, weight is another and physical constitution is another. Slight or frailer *vata*-like children require a smaller dose. Heavy or robust more *kapha*-like children can consume a larger dose. See the Ayurveda section on p211 for more information on *vata* and *kapha* characteristics.

Always use your intuition and their weight as guides. Clark's rule is very helpful here:

To determine the approximate dose for a child, divide the weight of the child in kilos by 75.

For example, for a child weighing 25kg, follow this sum 25 ÷ 75 = 0.33. Therefore the child's dose is ⅓ of the adult dose.

For a rule of thumb, these measures are also useful:

- 12 year-olds get an adult dose
- 6 year-olds get ½ an adult dose
- 3 year-olds get a ¼ adult dose
- Under 3 year-olds get just a few sips

What to drink tea from?

There is no 'right' cup or pot to make and drink herbal tea from. If you're brewing tea in a pot, then choose a sturdy one so it keeps your tea warm. The choice of cup is all yours… just make it beautiful. A good trick is to keep a lid on your cup when drinking aromatic herbs to prevent the valuable volatile oils from evaporating away.

Storing your herbs

The four enemies of all stored dried herbs are light, moisture, temperature and garlic. Keep them somewhere dark, dry, cool and away from strong smells. Hard roots and barks store for longer than delicate flowers and leaves. And everything stores better when kept somewhere airtight, cool and dark.

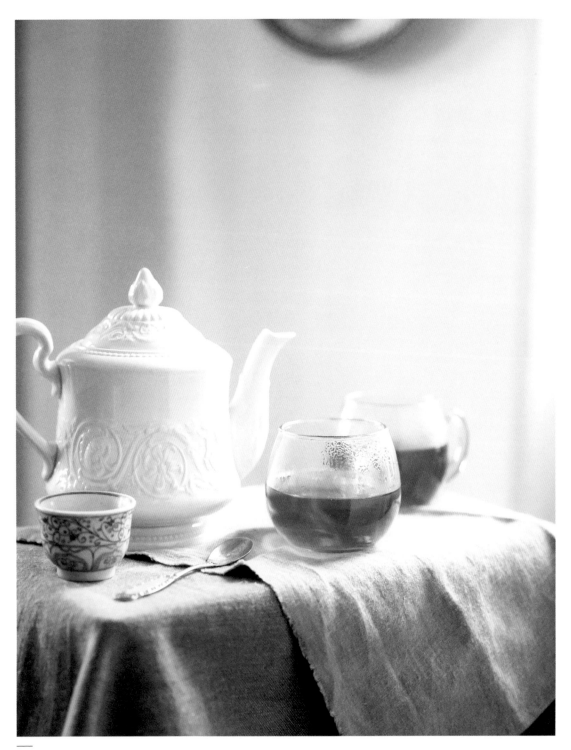

Helpful herbal terms

In herbal medicine special terms are used to describe how a plant works in the body, such as 'carminative', which means to calm digestive discomfort. Many of the terms originated in Western herbal medicine and are also commonly used in modern allopathic medicine. There are also terms used in Ayurveda that I've included, though you can find out more on this on p211.

Adaptogens are strengthening herbs that help us adapt to stress. They help normalise and nourish. Examples include ashwagandha root, shatavari and ginseng.

Alteratives are herbs that 'alter' the condition in a tissue by eliminating metabolic waste via the liver, large intestine, lungs, lymphatic system, skin and kidneys. Examples include burdock root, dandelion root and nettle leaf.

Amphoterics are herbs that bring balance to different organs, tissues and systems by regulating hyper and hypo functioning. Examples include licorice root, oat straw flowering tops and ashwagandha root.

Antimicrobials are herbs that interfere with the proliferation and life-cycle of microbes: bacteria, fungi and viruses. Examples include thyme leaf, echinacea and elderberry.

Aphrodisiac herbs are those that nourish, build and stimulate sexual desire and potency. Examples include shatavari, saffron and ashwagandha root.

Bile is secreted by the liver and stored in the gall-bladder. It helps us digest fats. It also helps stimulate bowel motions. If it coagulates it can form gall-stones.

Carminatives are high in essential oils and help ease digestion by relieving gas, spasms and cramps. Examples include aniseed, fennel seed and peppermint.

Demulcents are soothing mucilaginous and silky herbs that can be taken to soothe and protect damaged or inflamed tissue. Examples include slippery elm bark, marshmallow root and limeflower.

Diaphoretics are herbs that cause sweating by increasing circulation in the periphery of the body. Usually used to help relieve fevers. Examples include yarrow, elderflowers and ginger root.

Diuretics are herbs that stimulate the flow of urine and help remove fluids from the body. Examples include dandelion leaf, burdock root and corn silk.

Emmenagogues are herbs that stimulate and promote menstruation. Examples include turmeric root, marigold flowers and chaste tree berry fruits.

Expectorants are herbs that assist the body in expelling mucus from the upper respiratory tract. Examples include licorice root, elecampane root and thyme.

Galactagogues are herbs that encourage the flow of breastmilk. Examples include fennel seed, celery seed and shatavari.

Hepatics are herbs that support liver function. Examples include turmeric, dandelion root and yellow dock root.

Kapha is the Ayurvedic term for a specific constitutional type. It is responsible for stability and moisture and relates to the structure of the body. If kapha is out of balance then you may be overweight, have a heart problem, diabetes or high cholesterol. For more, see p211.

Laxative herbs are those that stimulate or promote bowel movements. There are different types: gentle aperients, like dandelion root; bulk-forming laxatives, like flax seed that increase the water and bulk of the stool; and stimulant laxatives like senna leaf that invigorate the muscles of the bowel to create a stronger motion.

Mucilage is a slippery, thick and viscous excretion from plants that is used to heal and soothe mucous membranes in the body. Marshmallow root, licorice root and aloe vera juice have abundant mucilage.

Nervines are herbs that soothe the nervous system and have a calming effect on the emotions. Examples include oat straw flowering tops, tulsi and passion flower.

Pitta is the Ayurvedic term for a specific constitutional type. It regulates heat and digestion and relates to metabolism and hormone production. If pitta is out of balance you may have heartburn, high blood pressure, skin rashes, hot flushes and be easily irritable. For more, see p211.

Tonics are herbs that bring tone to an organ or tissue, helping it to function better. It is also used to describe herbs that are general energy boosters. Examples include cacao, haritaki and amla.

Vata is the Ayurvedic term for a specific constitutional type. It regulates movement and communication and relates to the nervous system. If your vata is out of balance then you may suffer from insomnia, constipation, problem periods or infertility. For more, see p211.

Ailments & Elixirs

Acne
Help Me Glow (p36), Triphala Tea (p64)

ADHD
Cool Chamomile (p95), Pure Clarity (p99), Take It Easy (p104)

Adrenal Fatigue
Golden Milk Of Bliss (p73), Nourishing Nettle Tea (p74), Sweet Licorice (p127)

Alcohol/drug withdrawal
Pure Clarity (p99), Peace Tea (p100)

Allergies
Nourishing Nettle Tea (p74), Incredible Immunity (p148),

Alzheimer's
Pure Clarity (p99), Green Matcha Zen (p107)

Arthritis
Joint Protector (p154)

Asthma
Breathe (p138), Elderberry Elixir (p144)

Bleeding gums
Triphala Tea (p64)

Blood poisoning
I Love My Liver (p35), Help Me Glow (p36), Clean Greens (p196)

Blood pressure
Brave Heart (p123)

Blood sugar regulation
Natural Balance (p63)

Boils
I Love My Liver (p35), Help Me Glow (p36), Clean Greens (p196)

Breastfeeding
Golden Milk Of Bliss (p73), Mother's Milk (p169)

Bronchitis
Elderberry & Echinacea Winter Warmer (p140), Elderberry Elixir (p144)

Candida
Digestive Detox With A Twist (p39)

Catarrh
Ginger The Great (p52), Breathe (p138)

Chest infection
Ginger The Great (p52), Breathe (p138)

Chronic Fatigue Syndrome (CFS)
Golden Milk Of Bliss (p73), Heavenly Empress Vitality Tonic (p77), Sweet Licorice (p127)

Colds
Ginger The Great (p52), Breathe (p138), Lemon & Ginger With Manuka Honey (p147)

Constipation
A Good Move (p40), The Seeds Of Life (p193)

Cough
Breathe (p138)

Cystitis
Cool Waters (p45)

Depression
Melissa's Magic (p115), Let There Be Joy (p116), Bliss of The Gods (p124)

Dysmenorrhoea
Let There Be Joy (p116), Monthly Liberation (p175)

Eczema
Help Me Glow (p36), Clean Greens (p196)

Endometriosis
Moon Balance (p165), Monthly Liberation (p175)

Eyesight fatigue
Heavenly Empress Vitality Tonic (p77), Rise Like A Star (p89), Eagle Eyes (p151), Vitalise Berry Boost (p199)

Fertility
Golden Milk Of Bliss (p73), Heavenly Empress Vitality Tonic (p77), Aphrodite's Aphrodisiac (p162), The Seeds Of Life (p193)

Flatulence
Digestive Detox With A Twist (p39), A Good Move (p40), Take It Easy (p104), Digestive Lassi (p191)

Flu
Elderberry & Echinacea Winter Warmer (p140), Elderberry Elixir (p144), Incredible Immunity (p148)

Gout
Digestive Detox With A Twist (p39), Nourishing Nettle Tea (p74)

Haemorrhoids
Triphala Tea (p64), The Seeds Of Life (p193)

Hair loss
Heavenly Empress Vitality Tonic (p77), Illustriously Lustrous Locks (p153)

Halitosis
A Good Move (p40), Mint Digestif (p59)

Hayfever
Nourishing Nettle Tea (p74), Incredible Immunity (p148)

Heartburn
Fire Extinguisher (p60), Peppermint &
Licorice (p80)

Heart conditions
Brave Heart (p123)

Insomnia
Sweet Dreams (p103)

Irritable Bowel Syndrome (IBS)
Digestive Detox With A Twist (p39),
Majestic Mint (p56), Mint Digestif (p59)

Kidney health
A Royal Flush (p46)

Liver detox/problems
I Love My Liver (p35), Forgive Me
For I Have Sinned (p42)

Lung health
Sing A Song (p137), Elderberry Elixir
(p144), Lemon & Ginger With Manuka
Honey (p147)

Myalgic Encephalomyelitis (ME)
See Chronic Fatigue Syndrome

Menopause
Bliss of The Gods (p124), Cool Lady
(p170)

Migraine
Peace Tea (p100)

Mouth ulcer
I Love My Liver (p35)

Muscle strain/ache
Joint Protector (p154)

Obesity
Natural Balance (p63), Triphala Tea (p64)

Osteoporosis
Nourishing Almond Saffron Elixir (p70),
Heavenly Empress Vitality Tonic (p77)

Painful period
Monthly Liberation (p175)

Phlegm
Ginger The Great (p52), Breathe (p138),
Lemon & Ginger With Manuka Honey
(p147)

Piles
See haemorrhoids

Premenstrual Syndrome (PMS)
I Love My Liver (p35), Peace Tea (p100),
Moon Balance (p165)

Poly Cystic Ovarian Syndrome (PCOS)
Natural Balance (p63), Moon Balance
(p165)

Pregnancy
Nourishing Nettle Tea (p74), Full Moon
Celebrations (p166), Vitalise Berry
Boost (p199)

Prostate problems
Cool Waters (p45)

Psoriasis
I Love My Liver (p35), Help Me Glow
(p36), Triphala Tea (p64), Clean
Greens (p196)

Rash/hives
I Love My Liver (p35), Help Me Glow
(p36), Triphala Tea (p64), Clean
Greens (p196)

Reproductive health
Heavenly Empress Vitality Tonic (p77),
Aphrodite's Aphrodisiac (p162)

Restless Leg Syndrome (RLS)
Cool Chamomile (p95), Peace Tea (p100),
Take It Easy (p104)

Sinus problems
Ginger The Great (p52), Breathe (p138)

Skin
See eczema, acne, psoriasis

Sore throat
Elderberry & Echinacea Winter Warmer
(p140), Elderberry Elixir (p144)

Stomach acidity
See heartburn

Stress
Peace Tea (p100), Take It Easy (p104)

Tonsillitis
Elderberry & Echinacea Winter Warmer
(p140), Elderberry Elixir (p144)

Travel sickness
Ginger The Great (p52)

Urinary/bladder infection
Cool Waters (p45)

Water retention
Cool Waters (p45), Moon Balance (p165)

Weight loss
The Golden Ginger Triangle (p55), Natural
Balance (p63)

Women's health
I Love My Liver (p35), Heavenly Empress
Vitality Tonic (p77), Aphrodite's
Aphrodisiac (p162), Moon Balance (p165),

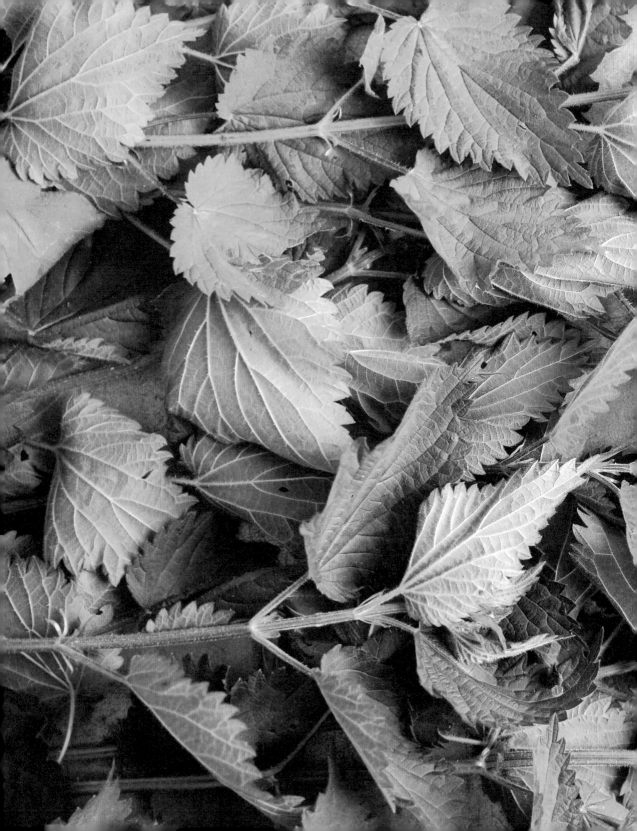

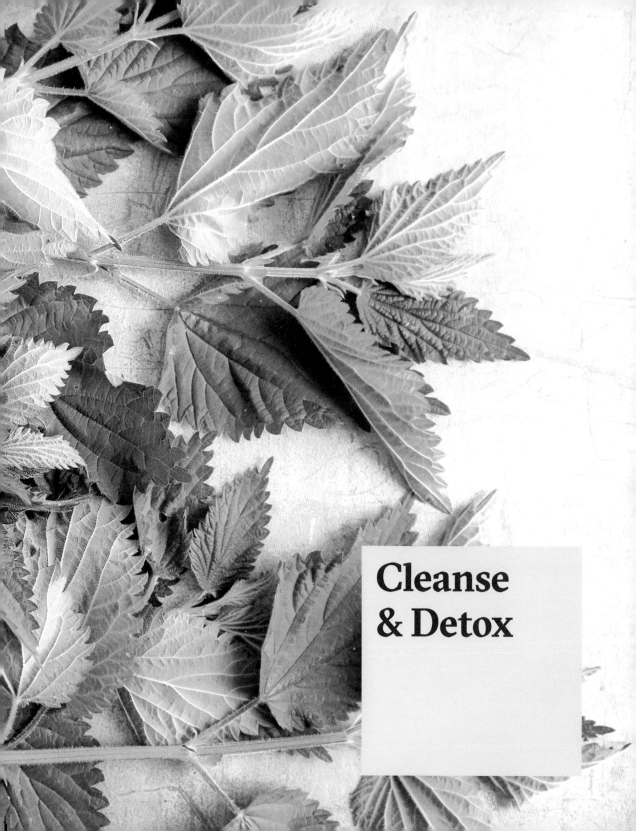

Cleanse
& Detox

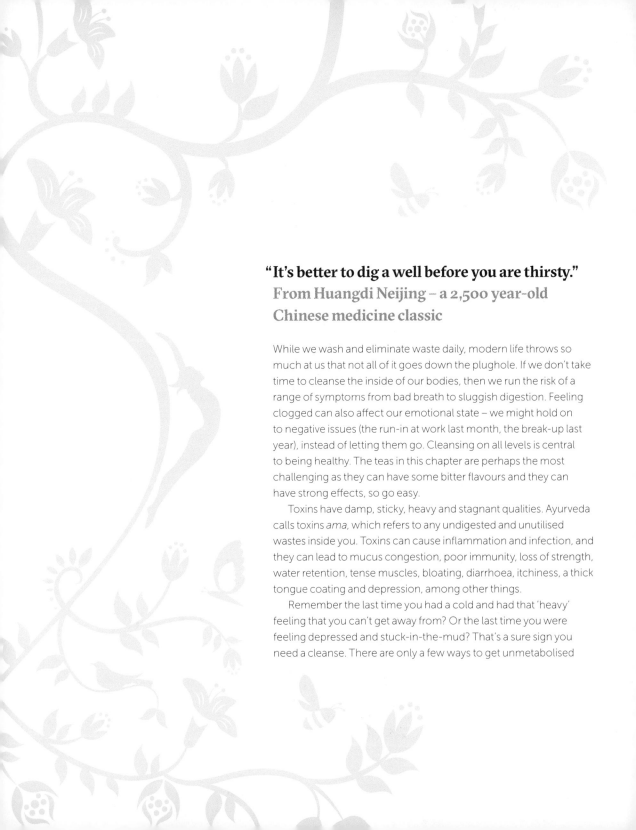

"It's better to dig a well before you are thirsty."
From Huangdi Neijing – a 2,500 year-old
Chinese medicine classic

While we wash and eliminate waste daily, modern life throws so much at us that not all of it goes down the plughole. If we don't take time to cleanse the inside of our bodies, then we run the risk of a range of symptoms from bad breath to sluggish digestion. Feeling clogged can also affect our emotional state – we might hold on to negative issues (the run-in at work last month, the break-up last year), instead of letting them go. Cleansing on all levels is central to being healthy. The teas in this chapter are perhaps the most challenging as they can have some bitter flavours and they can have strong effects, so go easy.

Toxins have damp, sticky, heavy and stagnant qualities. Ayurveda calls toxins *ama*, which refers to any undigested and unutilised wastes inside you. Toxins can cause inflammation and infection, and they can lead to mucus congestion, poor immunity, loss of strength, water retention, tense muscles, bloating, diarrhoea, itchiness, a thick tongue coating and depression, among other things.

Remember the last time you had a cold and had that 'heavy' feeling that you can't get away from? Or the last time you were feeling depressed and stuck-in-the-mud? That's a sure sign you need a cleanse. There are only a few ways to get unmetabolised wastes out of the body and these are what I rather graphically call The Six Ps: pee, poo, puke, perspiration, puffing (out of breath), pertussis (coughing) and, for women, periods. So our kidneys, bowels, lungs, skin and reproductive system are always helping us cleanse and maintain balance. And, of course, there is the liver. Every drug, artificial chemical, pesticide and hormone is broken down by enzyme pathways inside the liver cells. Many of the toxic chemicals that enter the body are fat soluble, which means they dissolve only in fatty or oily solutions and not in water. This makes them difficult for the body to excrete. Fat-soluble chemicals have a high affinity for fat tissues and cell membranes. In these fatty parts of the body, toxins may be stored for years, being released during times of exercise, stress or fasting. During the release of these toxins, symptoms such as headaches, nausea and fatigue may occur. The body's primary defence against toxins and poisons is provided by the liver. The liver is designed to convert fat-soluble chemicals into water-soluble chemicals so that they may then be easily excreted from the body via watery fluids such as bile and urine.

The best times of year to detox are at the junctions of the seasons (in March and September). While detoxification helps to refresh both body and mind, it is important that you nourish it properly afterwards. It's rather like weeding your garden then adding compost so that the flowers flourish. See the Energise & Rejuvenate chapter on p66 for the best nourishing teas.

For gram to teaspoon conversion see p24

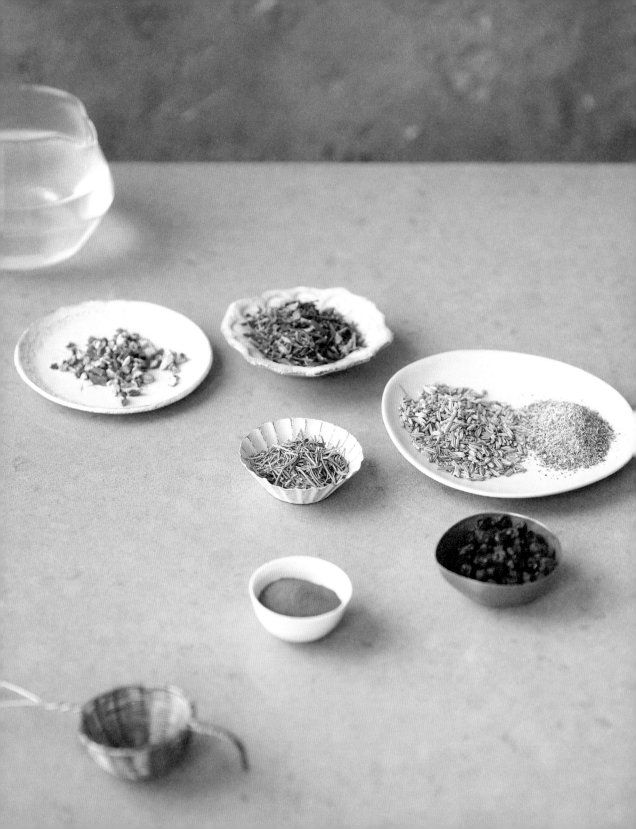

A beautifully bittersweet blend that helps to optimise your liver's health and happiness, restoring its vitality and tone. Our liver takes the brunt of the grunt work for metabolising wastes, so use this tea when you feel sluggish, your digestion is poor or you feel that you need a detox.

I love my liver

Dandelion root 4g
Schisandra berries 3g
Dandelion leaf 2g
Fennel seed 2g
Turmeric root powder 1g
Rosemary leaf 1g
Licorice root 1g

This will serve 2–3 cups of liver-loving tea.

Put all of the ingredients in a pot. Add 500ml/18fl oz freshly boiled filtered water. Leave to steep for 10–15 minutes, then strain.

If you want to really love your liver you could also try a little artichoke leaf, andrographis or neem, but they are not recommended in a tea as they are extremely bitter.

Dandelion root Slightly bittersweet, dandelion root is a cholagogue (stimulates bile flow), and it aids the liver and gall-bladder to remove any congestion and reduce inflammation.

Schisandra berries Known as the five-flavoured herb, this berry is a stalwart in Chinese herbal medicine that helps the liver metabolise toxins. It's brilliantly sweet and sour too.

Dandelion leaf Even more bitter than the root, dandelion leaf is a powerful diuretic and helps the liver flow.

Fennel seed Very sweet and full of *carminative* oils that relax your liver.

Turmeric root One of the all time great liver-loving herbs, turmeric root supports the organ's innate desire to clear the old and welcome the new.

Rosemary leaf Number one for moving stagnation and awakening the liver. Famous for removing fatty, sluggish and torpid liverish grumblings.

Licorice root A powerful liver-protector, licorice keeps the organ sweet and strong in the face of the many tasks it has to fulfil.

Cleanse & Detox

A healing blend of chlorophyll-rich herbs that purify the blood, soothe the liver and cleanse the skin, helping you glow from the inside out. Good for anyone with pimples, acne or other skin blemishes.

Help me glow

Nettle leaf 3g
Fennel seed 2g
Peppermint leaf 2g
Dandelion root 2g
Burdock root 2g
Red clover 2g
Turmeric root powder 1g
Licorice root 1g
Lemon juice a twist per cup

This will serve 2 cups of beautifying tea.

Put all of the ingredients in a pot (except the lemon). Add 500ml/18fl oz freshly boiled filtered water. Leave to steep for 10–15 minutes, then strain and add the lemon.

This recipe uses dry nettle, but you can collect your own fresh nettles in spring for a bright fresh tea. You can also dry the leaves for later use. Dry them on a plate or hang them somewhere cool for about a day.

Nettle leaf A blood cleanser par excellence. Nourishing, cleansing and rich in chlorophyll, nettle has been used for centuries as a skin purifier.

Fennel seed Renowned for preventing fermentation in your digestion and reducing the build up of inflammatory heat-toxins (these might show as spots or cystitis). Its gentle diuretic effects helps to flush out impurities.

Peppermint leaf Wonderfully aromatic, peppermint is famous for cooling the skin, calming an itch and reducing redness.

Dandelion root Slightly bittersweet, dandelion root helps the body to detoxify by enhancing the work of the liver and bowels.

Burdock root Earthy and powerful, burdock root is known as an *alterative*, working to cleanse your liver, kidneys and bowels. It's well-known for clearing facial blemishes.

Red clover Delicate and grassy, red clover blossom cleanses the skin and helps you glow.

Turmeric root Known as the Golden Goddess in India, turmeric is renowned for purifying the skin.

Licorice root This sweet root strengthens the kidneys and can help reduce skin inflammations.

Lemon juice This helps get your liver going in order to keep your skin clear and fresh.

Cleanse & Detox

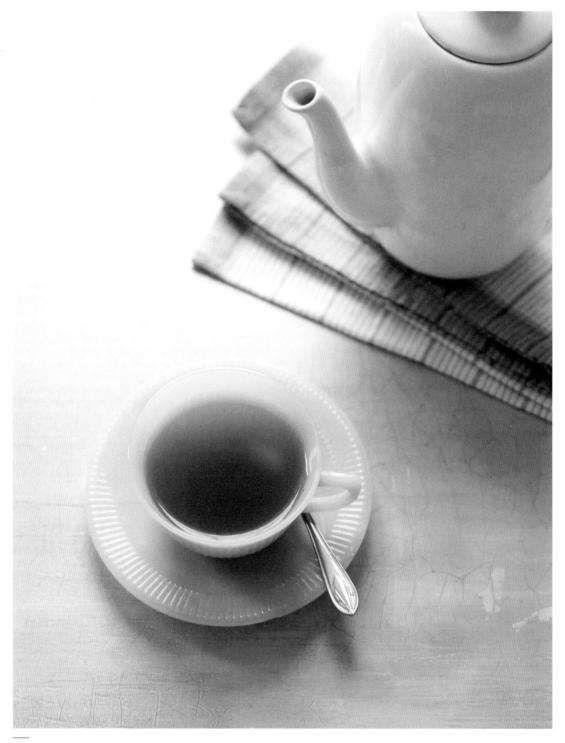

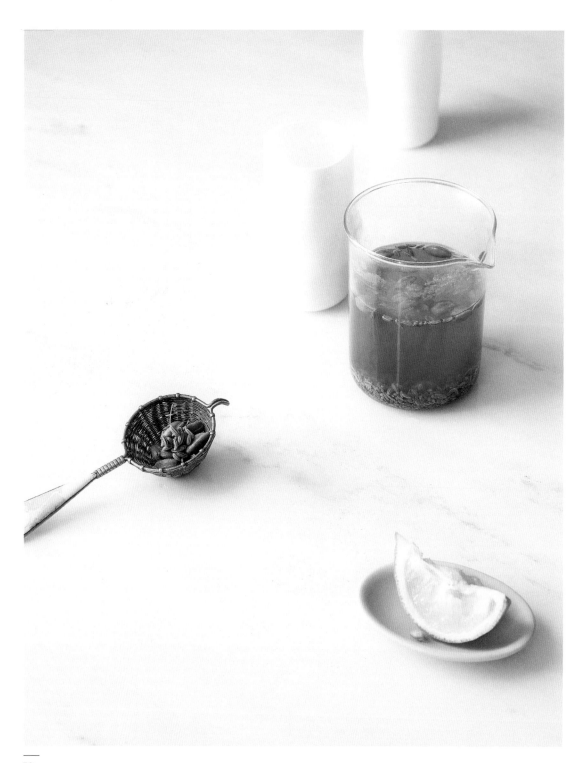

A detoxifying blend of tasty seeds and roots that help to regulate digestion, banish sluggishness and cleanse the blood. It's useful for anyone who gets bloated after eating.

Digestive detox with a twist

Aniseed 4g
Fennel seed 4g
Cardamom pod 3g
Dandelion root 2g
Licorice root 1g
Celery seed 1g
Lemon a twist per cup

This will serve 2 cups detoxifying tea with a citrus twist.

Put all of the ingredients in a pot (except for the lemon juice). Add 500ml/18fl oz freshly boiled filtered water. Leave to steep for 10–15 minutes, then strain. Enjoy with a twist of lemon in each cup.

This is a great tea to drink after a meal to help you get the best nourishment from your food and help you digest your meal more easily.

Aniseed Fragrant and sweet, this aromatic seed helps to clear wastes in the digestive system and lungs. Famed for clearing mucus and flushing the urinary system, it's an excellent detoxifier.

Fennel seed In Ayurveda, fennel seed balances all three constitutional types. It is great for soothing upset digestive systems and clears inflammatory toxins via the urinary tract.

Cardamom pod A warming *carminative*, this tropical seed-packed pod helps to clear toxins from the digestive system, blood and skin.

Dandelion root Slightly bittersweet, dandelion root supports the liver's detoxifying processes.

Licorice root This sweet root loves the kidneys and can help manage the effects of stress and the negative effects of excessive adrenaline by balancing the output of cortisol (steroid hormone). It is also an anti-inflammatory, helping to heal the skin inside and out.

Celery seed A very small but powerful seed that helps to clear uric acid from the blood and joints (high levels of uric acid can cause gout), and it strongly detoxifies the skin.

Lemon juice A twist of sweet and sour lemon juice helps your liver to release bile and metabolise waste more effectively.

A good move

There are only a few ways to move toxins out of the body – so if you're keen to cleanse, it's essential to make sure your bowels are working properly. This tea is one of the strongest of the lot, so proceed with caution. It will help you have a relaxed and cleansing bowel motion every day.

Yellow dock root 4g
Dandelion root 3g
Marshmallow root 2g
Senna leaf 2g
Orange peel 2g
Fennel seed 1g
Licorice root 1g

This will serve 2–3 cups of bowel-moving tea.

Put all of the ingredients in a pot. Add 500ml/18fl oz freshly boiled filtered water. Leave to steep for 10–15 minutes, then strain.

Just have 1 cup a day or you will find yourself trotting off to the loo too frequently. Don't use it for more than two weeks in a row as senna can cause some dependency. Make sure you keep properly hydrated throughout the day.

Whenever you eat a fresh organic orange, keep and dry the peel for a homemade stash of orange peel.

Yellow dock root A bittersweet gentle laxative that works by initiating the release of bile. Bile is the yellow stuff that helps to emulsify fats, making them more digestible. Yellow dock root also stimulates the bowel to move.

Dandelion root Its gentle and sweetening effect on the liver helps get the bowels going.

Marshmallow root Marshmallow root gives a soft, sweet and *demulcent* mucilage as it infuses in water – this can feel like an inner hug and helps to soothe as well as lubricate your digestive system.

Senna leaf An acrid-tasting herb that is strongly laxative, stimulating the bowel to move.

Orange peel This essential oil-packed peel tastes great and helps relax your digestive system so that the stronger herbs in this tea don't cause any griping pain.

Fennel seed Sweet and delightful, fennel seed freshens your whole system and helps alleviate tummy aches.

Licorice root Tastes great and counteracts the drying effects of the bitters while also adding a little lubricating effect to the blend.

Cleanse & Detox

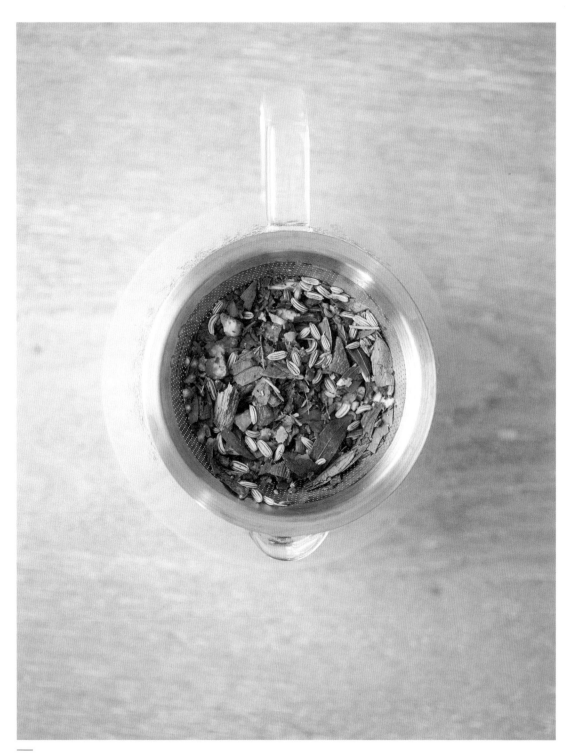

This is a help-you-feel-good tea to sip slowly after a night of indulgence. It aids digestion, stimulates sluggish circulation and refreshes your mind.

Forgive me for I have sinned

Fresh peppermint leaves
    1 handful (or 1 tbsp dry)
Fresh ginger root 3-5 slices
Fresh rosemary 2 sprigs
    (or 1 tsp dry)
Turmeric root powder ¼ tsp
    (or a sprinkle) per cup
Angostura bitters a dash per cup
Honey 1 tsp per cup

This will serve 2–3 cups of entirely confessional tea.

Put the mint, ginger and rosemary in a pot. Add 500ml/18fl oz freshly boiled filtered water. Leave to steep for 10–15 minutes, then strain. Add the turmeric, bitters and honey. Breathe in the aromas while you drink this, they will help you feel better.

Peppermint leaf Like a good friend, peppermint is always welcome. Its light ascendant menthol awakens digestion and clears sluggishness. It can encourage a fresh perspective when things seem to be blocking your way.

Ginger root Considered to be good for everybody, fresh ginger moves your energy upwards and outwards waking up your whole system. Its sweet-spicy nature diffuses any clouds obscuring your view.

Rosemary Better on its own than you might think, rosemary is famous for helping you think more clearly by removing a muzzy head. It literally pulls you up by your socks.

Turmeric root A renowned liver cleanser, turmeric speeds up the metabolism of alcohol and fats, making your day a whole lot easier, a whole lot faster.

Angostura bitters A classic herbal concoction. A dash of these super herbs can awaken your digestion and transport you to another world (far away from your hangover).

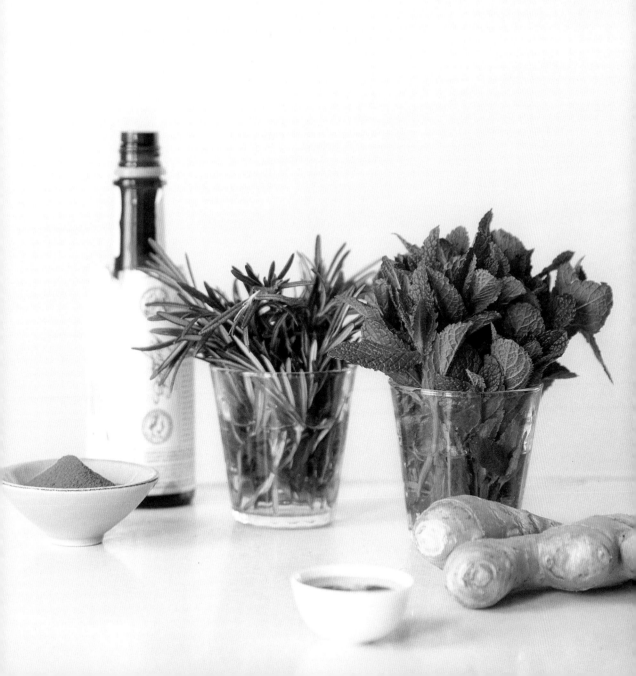

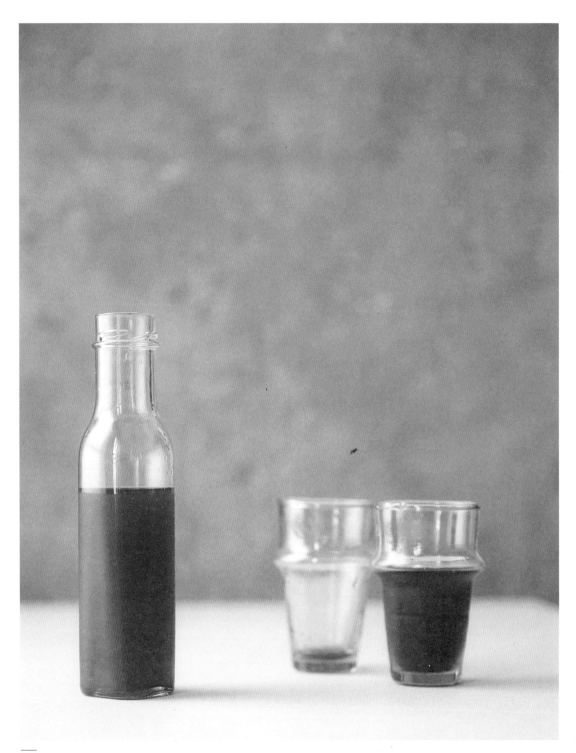

Cool waters

If you ever suffer from urinary tract infections, then this is the tea for you. It helps to soothe the bladder and gets your golden stream flowing with ease. As the saying goes: 'it's better to dig a well before you're thirsty' – so keep these ingredients on hand as part of your 'green' first aid kit.

Marshmallow root 4g
Coriander seed 4g
Buchu leaf 5g
Uva ursi leaf 5g
Corn silk 4g
Dandelion leaf 3g
Cranberry juice 1 tsp concentrate
     (or 50ml/2fl oz juice) per cup

This will serve 2 cups of definitely diuretic tea.

Put the marshmallow root and coriander seeds in a pot. Add 200ml/7fl oz cold water and leave overnight (their urinary-soothing mucilage is best extracted in cold water). The next day put the rest of the ingredients (except for the cranberry juice) in another pot. Add 400ml/14fl oz freshly boiled filtered water and leave to steep for 20–30 minutes. Strain, then combine the two liquids. Add the cranberry concentrate or juice to each cup of tea. This is good served cold too.

A little sodium bicarbonate can be used every day to alkalise acidic urine. Add ½ tsp to water and drink it with this tea.

Marshmallow root This silky-sweet herb softens any irritation and soothes the flow of fluids throughout the urinary system.
Coriander seed Sweet and aromatic, coriander seed is a favourite remedy for clearing heat from urinary channels, which is particularly helpful if you suffer from cystitis.
Buchu leaf The buchu leaf has renowned antimicrobial qualities that also tone the urinary system.
Uva ursi leaf Famous for restoring the ecology of the urinary system, it can act as a potent antimicrobial and astringent helping to soothe and relieve any pain.
Corn silk This is the golden hairs from inside the sheath of a fresh corn on the cob – it is one of nature's most effective diuretics. Corn silk really makes you pee more, helping to flush the system. (You can collect corn silk whenever you eat corn on the cob and dry it to use in your tea.)
Dandelion leaf Known as *pis en lit* (French for 'wet the bed'), dandelion leaf is a fantastic diuretic. It is brimming with potassium, meaning it can drain fluids while balancing sodium-potassium levels so you don't get dehydrated.
Cranberry juice Try to find a cranberry juice concentrate or juice without sugar – it will freshen the tea. The water-loving red fruit is antimicrobial and can aid the tone of the urinary system.

Our kidneys are a wonder of nature's intricate design. Its vital roles include filtering blood, maintaining electrolyte balance and regulating blood pressure, as well as balancing mineral levels and acid-alkaline ratios. This is a gentle tea that can flush your kidneys, help prevent gravel accumulating and remove fluid congestion. Don't drink it before bed or you will be up all night visiting the bathroom. And if you actually have a kidney stone see your doctor and a herbalist before using this tea.

A royal flush

Plantain leaf 3g
Goldenrod flowering top 3g
Gokshura seed 3g
Burdock root 3g
Marshmallow root 2g
Fennel seed 2g

This will serve 2 cups of kidney-cleansing tea.

Put all of the ingredients in a pot. Add 500ml/18fl oz of freshly boiled filtered water. Leave to steep for 20–30 minutes, then strain.

Plantain leaf This ubiquitous and often trampled on herb directs this tea to the kidneys and is an excellent diuretic.

Goldenrod flowering top This brilliant yellow flower helps to clean the pipes and works to clear gravel from the complex kidney network.

Gokshura seed Often referred to by its Latin name *Tribulus terrestris*, this is one of the spikiest herbs in the world so handle with caution. Their pointed barbs are said to metaphorically 'scrape' stones from the system. Gokshura seed is a potent kidney tonic used to generally enhance muscle mass and bring strength.

Burdock root A favourite *alterative* herb that balances kidney function and makes us pee.

Marshmallow root It could be called marsh*mellow* root as it's so soothing to irritations.

Fennel seed A simple diuretic that helps to sweeten the tea and ease your pee.

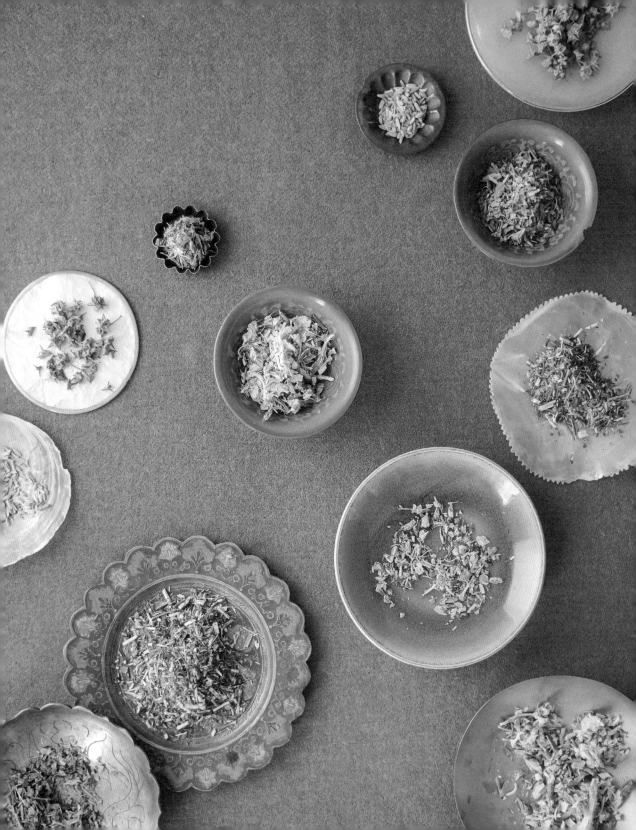

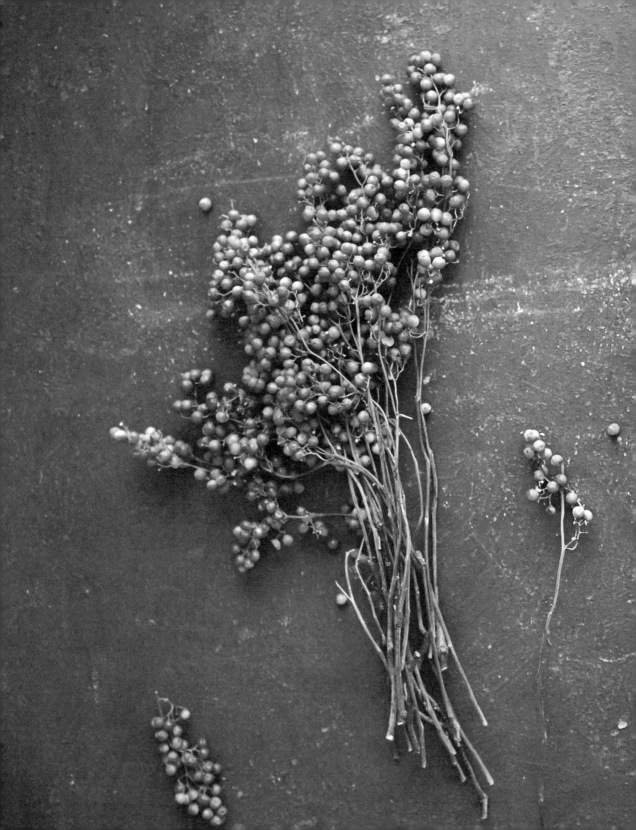

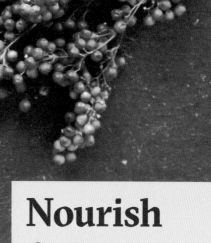

Nourish
& Digest

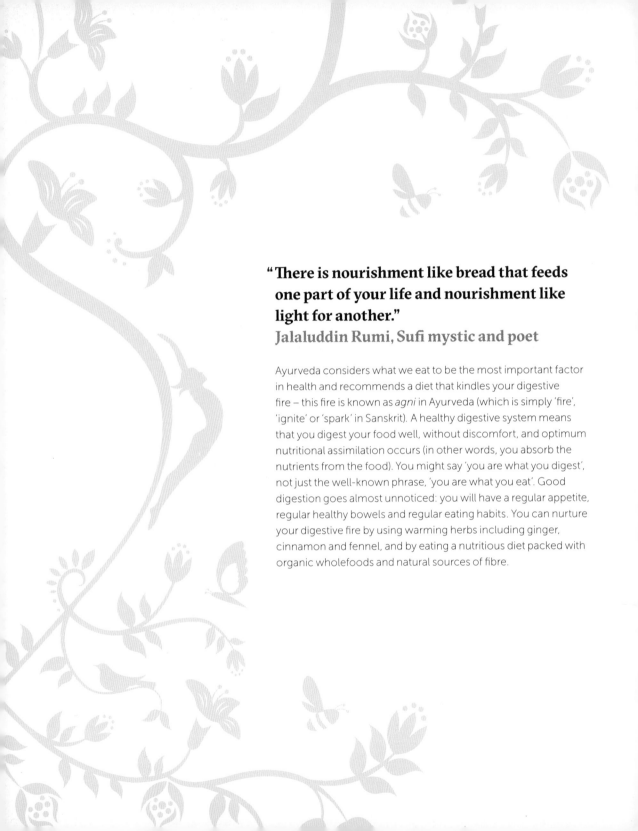

"There is nourishment like bread that feeds
one part of your life and nourishment like
light for another."
Jalaluddin Rumi, Sufi mystic and poet

Ayurveda considers what we eat to be the most important factor
in health and recommends a diet that kindles your digestive
fire – this fire is known as *agni* in Ayurveda (which is simply 'fire',
'ignite' or 'spark' in Sanskrit). A healthy digestive system means
that you digest your food well, without discomfort, and optimum
nutritional assimilation occurs (in other words, you absorb the
nutrients from the food). You might say 'you are what you digest',
not just the well-known phrase, 'you are what you eat'. Good
digestion goes almost unnoticed: you will have a regular appetite,
regular healthy bowels and regular eating habits. You can nurture
your digestive fire by using warming herbs including ginger,
cinnamon and fennel, and by eating a nutritious diet packed with
organic wholefoods and natural sources of fibre.

Five steps to digestive peace

The majority of your diet should be freshly cooked,
eaten warm and made with spices that aid digestion.

1. Warm drinks nurture your digestive fire.
2. Cold drinks kill it.
3. Remember your stomach is about the size of your
   cupped hands and it's best to keep portions in line
   with this to help you have an easy day.
4. Wait until you have fully digested your previous meal
   before you eat again and try not to eat on the go –
   your digestion works best when you are relaxed.
5. Follow your gut instinct and most importantly,
   enjoy your food.

If you follow these five steps 90 per cent of the time you'll be
well on your way to good digestive health. Of course, herbal
teas would be included in a list of the best ways to nurture your
digestion. They can pick it up, get it moving, slow it down and
help it work better in whatever way you need.

For gram to teaspoon
conversion see p24

Ginger the great

Probably the best tea of all, it reaches parts of the body that other herbal teas just can't reach. I use it to wake up my digestive system, warm me up and help me be present in the moment. Ginger is my go-to herb whenever I feel a chill wind blowing.

Fresh ginger root 5g, about 2.5cm/1in

This will serve 1 cup of warming ginger tea.

Scrub the ginger or lightly peel. If you choose to peel ginger, use a teaspoon to scrape the skin away (it's the best way by far – granny's top tip).

Slice the ginger into fine slivers and put in a pot. Add 250ml/9fl oz of freshly boiled filtered water. Leave to steep for 10–15 minutes. You can then strain it, or you can leave the ginger in. If you want to make the tea stronger, you can simmer the ginger in a pan with the lid on for a few minutes.

Ginger root Digestion's best friend, ginger is warming and spicy with thermogenic properties that increase metabolism. Its spiciness is not only delicious but also helps us to absorb more nutrients from our food.

It contains the wonderfully named gingerols and shogaols – these natural plant-protectors have been shown to stimulate the circulation and reduce the stickiness of our platelets to give our blood a healthier profile. Shogaols in particular have antiemetic properties, helping to relieve nausea.

In Ayurveda, ginger is known as the 'universal medicine' which is good for everyone. It's easy to see why, as it's regarded as an excellent *carminative* (a herb that reduces intestinal gas) and an intestinal spasmolytic (a herb that relaxes and soothes the intestinal tract). Its ability to penetrate deeply into the body helps it to relieve stiffness and pain and it's commonly used as a powerful antioxidant and anti-inflammatory for arthritis. Fresh ginger also encourages peripheral circulation, warming the tips of your fingers and toes (while dry ginger is more warming to your core). Ginger thrives in the hot Asian sun, absorbing its potent heat and then offering it to us whenever we need warming up.

If you have any pain on your body you can make a flannel soak with this tea. Make the tea, soak a flannel in the hot infusion, ring out any excess fluids and apply to the area. I use this at the first sign of a sore throat and apply to the chest and throat until the skin is reddened, or use it to soothe painful joints or muscles. A flannel soak is also useful for reducing period pain – just place the hot ginger-tea soaked flannel over the painful area.

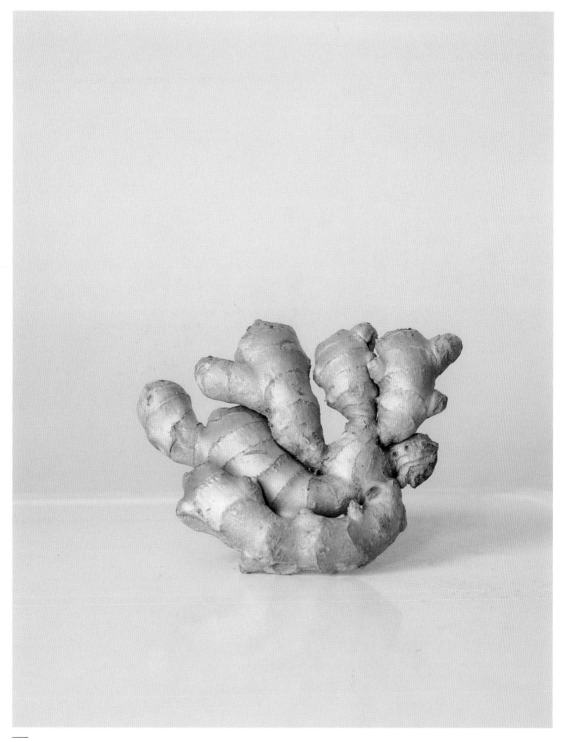

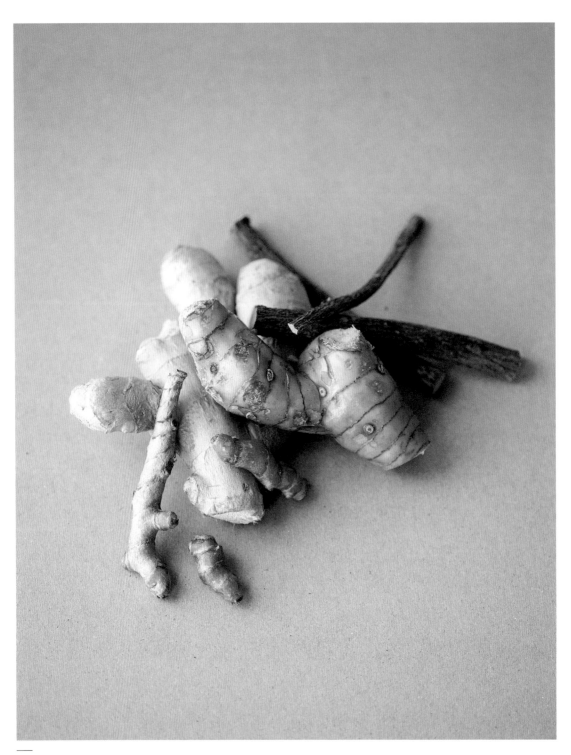

This trio are members of the *Zingiberaceae* (ginger) family – together they make a potent tea full of warmth. Surviving in hot and humid jungles, these three are familiar with warding off damp – so they should also keep you feeling fresh. If you have a sluggish metabolism, drink this tea daily.

The golden ginger triangle

Fresh ginger root 4g, about 2cm/¾in
   (or 2g dry)
Fresh galangal root 2g, about 1cm/½in
   (or 1g dry)
Fresh turmeric root 2g, about 1cm/½in
   (or 1g dry)
Licorice root 2g

This will serve 2–3 cups of golden tea.

Put all of the ingredients in a pot. Add 500ml/18fl oz of freshly boiled filtered water. Leave to steep for 10–15 minutes, then strain. If you want to make the tea stronger you can simmer it in a pan with the lid on for a few minutes.

Ginger root This is wonderfully warming to your core. It improves digestion, increases circulation and tastes good too.
Galangal root Galangal might transport you to a tropical realm with its sweet and fragrant qualities. Commonly used in Asian cooking, it has similar properties to ginger root and, among other things, is also a good friend to the lungs, helping to strengthen them and clear coughs and mucus.
Turmeric root Ginger's more showy sister, turmeric is the most beautiful hue of golden-yellow and adds a bit of vibrant colour to life. Turmeric really is good for just about everything from immunity to metabolism. It has a slightly earthy flavour and its lemony notes blend well with ginger and galangal.
Licorice root Sweet and mellow, licorice is a nourishing tonic for the nervous system, adrenals, lungs and digestion. It helps to balance some of the extreme fiery heat of the gingers in this tea.

Nourish & Digest

Majestic mint

This is a wake-up in a cup. Fresh, uplifting and enlivening, this blend of refreshing mints will assist your digestive system and awaken your mind. Drinking a mild cup of hot mint tea (made with a two grams of dry mint or a sprig of fresh) helps you to relax and feel 'in yourself', and is especially settling for upset digestion. Drinking a strong cup of hot mint tea (five of more grams of dry mint or a big handful of fresh leaves) is stimulating and sends your energy to the periphery of your body (head, fingers, toes and skin). This is a simple go-to remedy if you have a winter bug as it is a mild *diaphoretic* that can induce a gentle sweat and help to relax any muscle tension.

As many types of fresh mint as you can find (try peppermint, spearmint, horsemint and fieldmint) 10–20g, about 2 handfuls

This will serve 2–3 cups of minty tea.

Put all of the ingredients in a pot. Add 500ml/18fl oz of freshly boiled filtered water. Leave to steep for 5–10 minutes, then strain. Some people like a little sweetener with the mint – honey works a treat.

Peppermint A hybrid of spearmint and watermint and, after green tea, the most popular herbal tea in the world.
Spearmint A classic Moroccan mint that is slightly sweeter and less intense than peppermint or fieldmint.

All mints are brimming with an array of tasty and therapeutic essential oils. Fieldmint contains the largest amount of these essential oils by a long way. It's the mint used for extracting the menthol flavourings and is added to many of our mint-flavoured foods. These mints are strong aromatic *carminatives* and decongestants, and they help to ease a sluggishness in the digestive system or lungs. You can experience an 'opening' effect when you smell any mint – breathe in deeply and feel your senses awaken and your mind light up.

Nourish & Digest

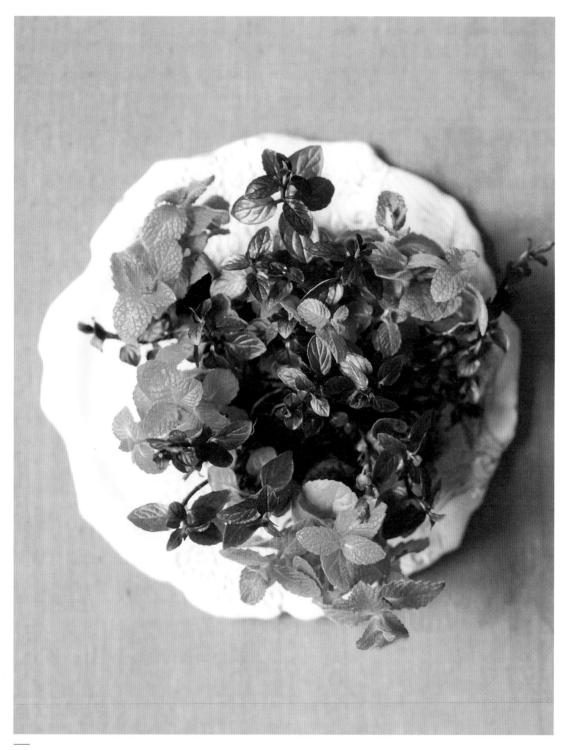

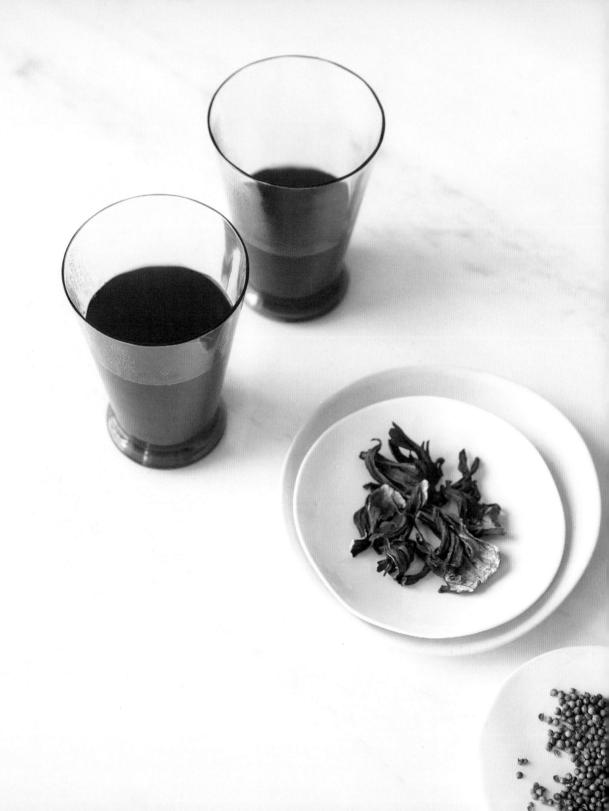

There is an Ayurvedic saying: 'all disease starts with poor digestion'. This tea will help boost your digestive fire without over-heating it. It is a *pitta*-balancing tea made for sipping after a sumptuous meal.

Mint digestif

Peppermint leaf 4g
Licorice root 2g
Hibiscus flower 2g
Fennel seed 1g
Coriander seed 1g

This will serve 2–3 cups of a delicious digestif tea.

Put all of the ingredients in a pot. Add 500ml/18fl oz of freshly boiled filtered water. Leave to steep for 5–10 minutes, then strain.

Peppermint leaf This aromatic leaf prevents spasms and pain in the digestive tract. Its menthol is also wonderfully cooling to any excess acid in the stomach. It has a spreading and opening function that helps to ease any post-meal bloating.

Licorice root A great herb for moderating digestive irritation as it is soothing and relaxing. A specific for sweetening excess acidity in the digestive system.

Hibiscus flower The beautiful hibiscus is mildly sweet and sour and helps to support the digestive process after a rich meal.

Fennel seed Great for settling an unhappy digestive system, fennel seed's essential oils are powerfully antispasmodic, helping to calm digestion and assist in the body's absorption of nutrients. In Ayurveda, fennel seed balances all three constitutional types.

Coriander seed This seed is especially good for strong digestion, but doesn't over-stimulate the system.

As the name suggests, this tea is purely functional – its aim is to clear acid and rebalance an over-acidic digestive system. When heat accumulates in the system it can cause heartburn or an upset stomach, and these herbs quickly extinguish the flames.

Fire extinguisher

Meadowsweet leaf 3g
Marshmallow leaf 2g
Peppermint leaf 2g
Chamomile flower 2g
Rose flower 1g
Licorice root 1g
Slippery elm bark powder ½ tsp per cup (please note this is a threatened species so only buy from a verified sustainable and organic source)
Aloe vera juice a glug (or 1 tbsp) per cup

This will serve 2–3 cups of heartburn-extinguishing tea.

Put all of the ingredients in a pot (except for the slippery elm bark and aloe vera juice). Add 500ml/18fl oz of freshly boiled filtered water. Leave to steep for 1 hour, then strain. Allow to cool. Stir ½ tsp of slippery elm powder and a glug of aloe vera juice into each cup of cool tea before drinking cold.

Meadowsweet leaf Known as the Queen of the Meadow, meadowsweet is astringent and is specific for heartburn and indigestion caused by acidity. It's not the best-tasting herb in the world, but it has a brilliant effect.

Marshmallow leaf Soft like velvet, marshmallow leaf soothes irritated and burning digestive systems.

Peppermint leaf Just a pinch of peppermint leaf brings instant cooling to a burning digestive fire.

Chamomile flower Slightly bitter, these bright yellow buds help ease any inflammation in your stomach.

Rose flower The perfect remedy for calming agitated heartburn. Rose petals also help bring peace to any emotional problems that might be upsetting your tummy.

Licorice root Its silky soothing qualities clear acid while its sweetness calms irritation from digestive pain. It also counteracts any bitterness in the other herbs in this tea.

Slippery elm bark powder A true *demulcent* containing mucilage that coats mucous membranes in the gut, helping to protect and heal from any burning fire.

Aloe vera juice This is the icing on the cake: cooling, healing and a perfect elixir for heartburn.

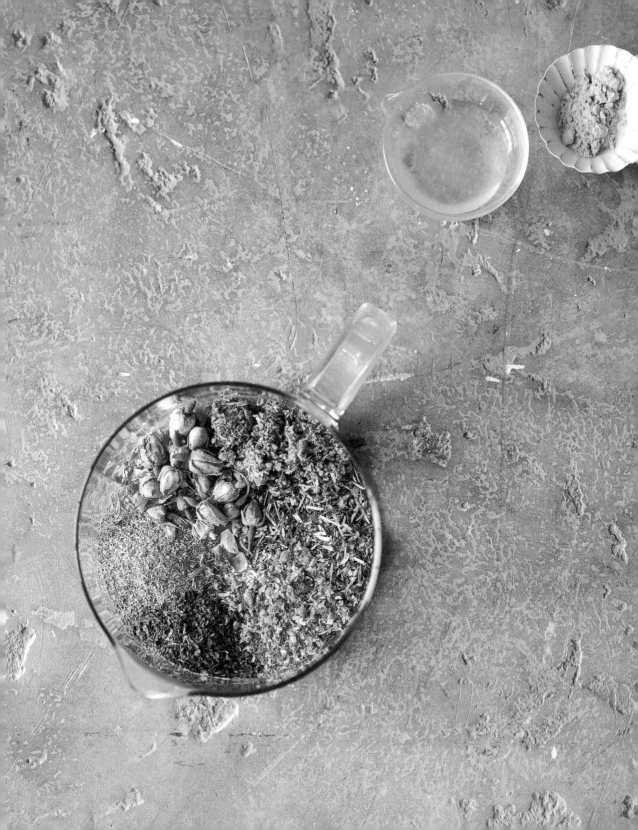

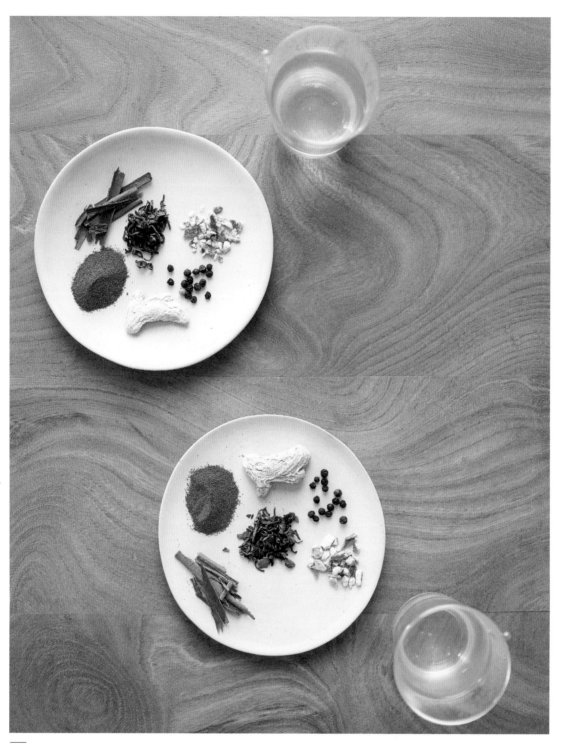

Natural balance

When our digestive fire is low it cannot transform food into nourishing energy. Instead food can get stored as fat, starting a vicious cycle where digestion becomes weaker and weaker, leading to steady weight gain. This tea stimulates metabolism to help you find your natural and balanced weight. It's a fiery one.

Cinnamon bark 4g
Ginger root powder 2g
Orange peel 2g
Green tea 2g
Turmeric root powder 1g
Black pepper 1g
Orange essential oil a drop per cup

This will serve 2–3 cups of digestion-enhancing, weight-balancing tea that works together with lots of exercise.

Put all of the ingredients in a pot (except for the orange essential oil). Add 500ml/18fl oz freshly boiled filtered water. Leave to steep for 10–15 minutes, then strain. Add one drop of orange essential oil to each cup.

Cinnamon bark Hot, warming, sweet and astringent, cinnamon boosts the metabolism. It specifically helps with regulating sugar levels so that any insulin-resistance does not lead to fat storage. It also reduces total cholesterol. It's my go-to for finding a balanced and healthy weight.

Ginger root Spicy and stimulating, ginger root boosts strength in the digestive system and helps the metabolism work more efficiently.

Orange peel According to the doctrine of signatures (see p15), orange peel's appearance hints at its effects – i.e. it's good for cellulite. Its warming properties help boost digestion and metabolism. Adding orange essential oil helps to awaken digestive function and clear sluggishness.

Green tea An excellent thermogenic herb that ignites your life-force, green tea helps to metabolise fat.

Turmeric root Long used for enhancing the digestive process and helping reduce obesity, turmeric has recently been shown to promote a healthy body fat percentage.

Black pepper Rocket fuel for the metabolism.

For an extra boost for your digestive system, drink Triphala Tea (on p64), as well as Natural Balance.

Now this is a strange one. It's not really a normal tea – it's more of a cold infusion used in Ayurveda as a digestive and rejuvenating aid. It has a rather, shall we say 'therapeutic' astringent flavour, but it's pleasantly sour and sweet too.

Triphala tea

Triphala powder 1–3g, about 1 tsp

This will serve 1 cup of healing tea.

Put the triphala powder in a glass and add 200ml/7fl oz cold water. Cover and leave overnight. (For a truly cosmic experience, place the glass in moonlight.) The next morning drink the liquid for a refreshing start to the day.

Triphala Ayurveda's most famous formula is made from equal parts of three fruits: haritaki, bibhitaki and amla. It helps to detoxify and to nourish and is traditionally used to maintain a healthy digestive tract. Use triphala when there are signs of sluggish bowels, constipation, bloating, flatulence, abdominal pain and indigestion. It can help to heal ulcers, reduce inflammation, heal haemorrhoids and aid microbial imbalance in the gastro-intestinal tract. If you are regularly constipated use it with some psyllium husks to bring some moisture into your bowels. As a toxin digester, it helps to clear a furry tongue and fermenting bowel; as an appetiser it promotes a healthy desire for food; as a blood cleanser it reduces skin blemishes; and as a mild laxative it banishes constipation without causing dependency. It redirects the flow of energy downwards, helping to regulate your motions. It is an overall rejuvenative, considered to prolong life.

Just 2g of triphala has potent antioxidant activity higher than a whole cup of cherries.

Nourish & Digest

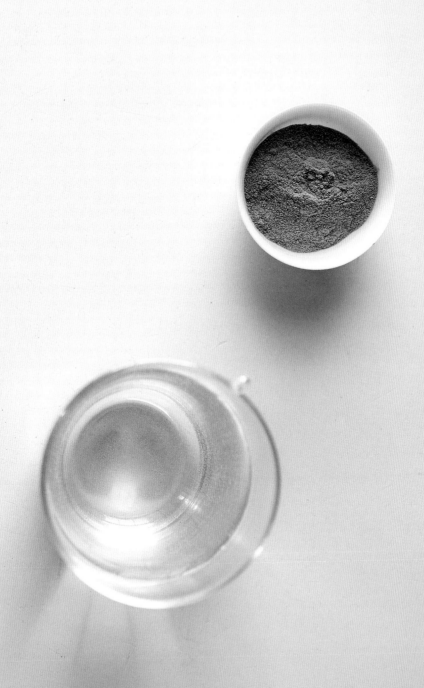

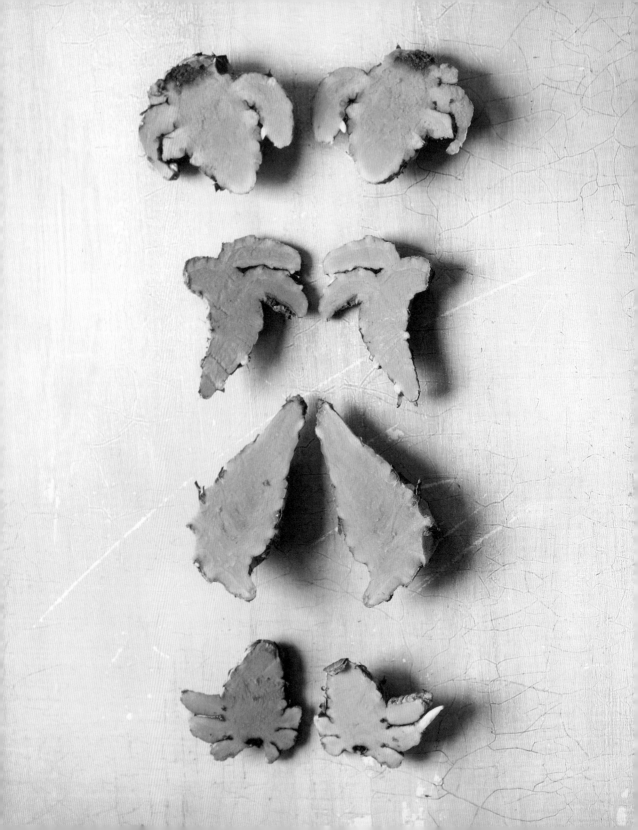

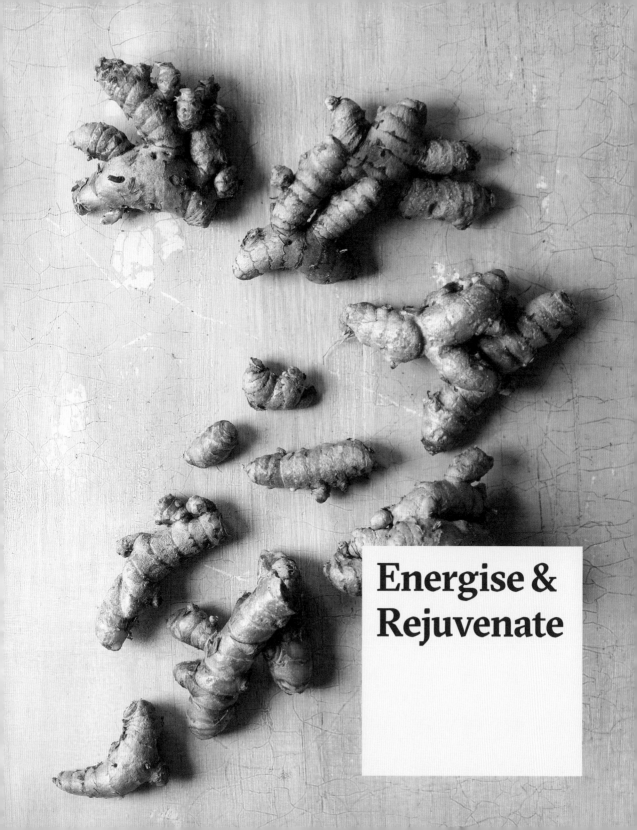

Energise &
Rejuvenate

"Rejuvenation brings you a long life, a sharp memory, intelligence, freedom from disease, youthfulness, beauty, a sweet voice, respect and brilliance."
Ayurveda doctor Charaka, from Charaka Samhita written some 2,000 years ago

Rejuvenation is as important as cleansing and nourishing. It helps bring joy and vitality to life. Ayurveda calls rejuvenation *rasayana*. *Rasa* means 'juicy' and *ayana* means 'extending' – extending our juice – so rejuvenation is about increasing both the quality and quantity of the juiciness, satisfaction and enjoyment of life.

Just imagine feeling full of energy, bursting with vitality, having bright eyes, clear skin, a quick healing response, healthy desires and being full of optimism. That's rejuvenation brimming with energy.

Life is more difficult when we don't feel our best. Health is wealth, and the best way to be healthy is to be constantly renewing and replenishing body and mind. Rejuvenation hastens recovery from disease, it improves your mind and intellect and it promotes longevity and delays the signs of ageing. We need to consistently rejuvenate because the opposite of this is to forever be operating under par.

As the majority of health imbalances come from some sort of

deficiency or weakness, when you get run down this invariably affects your immunity. When you have a 'deficiency' you can feel tired, stressed and look washed-out. It's the natural result of living a busy life where you give out more than you get back. It happens to all of us, but the trick is knowing how to replenish. In essence, you need to reverse this process of decline with regular top-ups of rejuvenation. This can be a holiday, a yoga class, a massage or time with friends and family. You can also optimise your energy on a daily basis by regulating your lifestyle, diet and herbs.

My favourite ways to rejuvenate are yoga, breathing and, of course, a good cup of herbal tea. A colourful diet, massage and being in love are also extremely boosting but, as this is a book about herbal teas, let's talk about some herbs.

Think of rejuvenating herbs as special micro-nutrient-tonics for supporting your wellness. Herbs like ginseng, ashwagandha and shatavari are world-famous rejuvenators. An amazing feature of most rejuvenating herbs is their ability to help us adapt to stress, hence many of them are known as *adaptogens*. They often grow in extreme climates where they acquire the energy to adjust to a stressful environment. Their excellence manifests from their non-specific nature: *adaptogens* are proficient generalists. They perform multiple actions on diverse organ and tissue systems at the same time. Sometimes they nudge us, sometimes they push us, but they always support us.

For gram to teaspoon
conversion see p24

This is heaven in a glass. Golden, silken and sweet, it builds your brain and your brawn.

Nourishing almond saffron elixir

Almonds 10
Saffron 5 strands
Cardamom seed from 1–2 pods
Water 150ml/5¼fl oz
Honey to taste

This will serve 1 cup of nourishing tea.

Soak the 10 almonds overnight. The next day, squeeze/peel the outer skin off the nuts. Put the skinless nuts in a blender with the saffron, cardamom seeds and water, and whizz until combined. Add honey to taste. Drink first thing in the morning for an early experience of joy.

Almonds Considered in Ayurveda to be a rejuvenative par excellence, this nutrient-dense nut nourishes the deep tissues of the reproductive, nervous and bone systems, promoting strength and vitality. Soaking the almonds overnight brings them alive, so they are sprouting with enzymatic life.

Saffron This delicate beauty is brimming with the essence of life. It is a renowned rejuvenator, uplifting the spirits and reaching deep into the body to act as an ambrosial aphrodisiac for both men and women.

Cardamom seed Cardamom's ethereal aroma lifts sluggishness and helps to awaken the digestive system and the mind.

Honey Nature's elixir, honey helps to bring pleasure, energy and a sense of satisfaction.

Energise & Rejuvenate

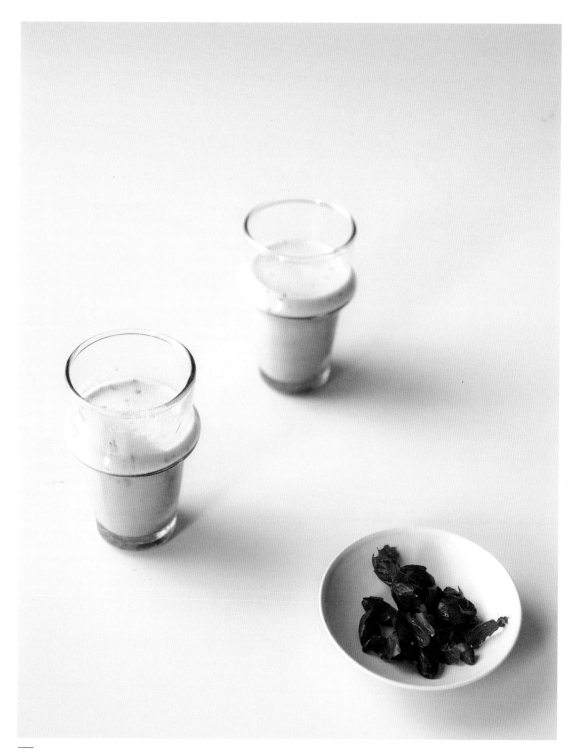

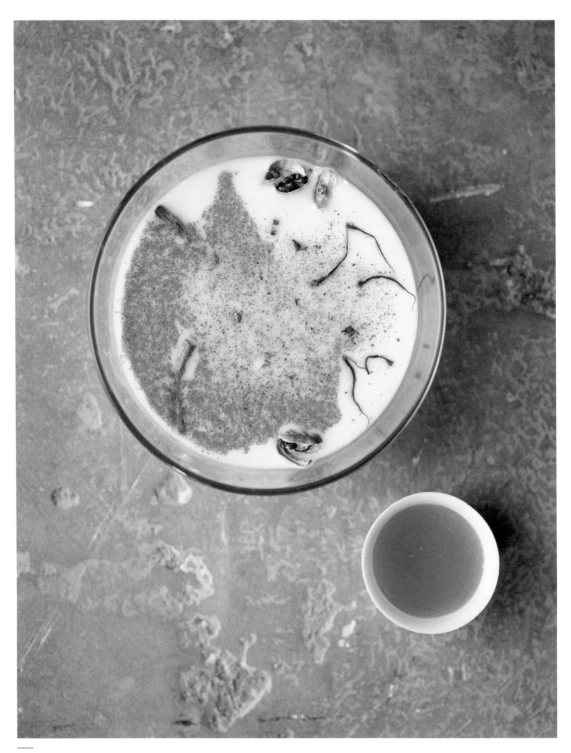

A warm nectar to nourish you deep inside. It helps to replenish your nervous and sexual energies. It is literally bliss in a cup. It's a great relaxant so drink this one warm before bed. This has all the benefits of Nourishing Almond Saffron Elixir (p70), but with the deeper calming properties of warm milk, nutmeg and ashwagandha.

Golden milk of bliss

Almond, rice or other milk 150ml/
   5¼fl oz
Ground almond 2 tsp
Cardamom pod 2 pods (gently
   crushed/split)
Saffron 5 strands
Turmeric root powder a pinch
Nutmeg powder a pinch
Ashwagandha root ¼ tsp
Honey to taste

This will serve 1 cup of blissful tea.

Gently warm the milk in a pan for a few minutes, then add the rest of the ingredients (except for the honey). Pour into a cup and stir in some honey. (Ashwagandha powder has a bit of a funny taste, so if you prefer you can take an ashwagandha capsule when you drink the milk instead.) The ground almond sinks to the bottom, so stir before drinking.

Almond This delicious nut is sweet to taste, heating, heavy and oily in quality. It builds, strengthens and has aphrodisiac qualities that boost fertility.

Cardamom pod The aromatic essential oils in cardamom are used to help digest the highly nutritious fats in this replenishing elixir.

Saffron One of the remarkable things about saffron is that the colourful pigments are both water- and fat-soluble meaning its depression-lifting, blood-circulating, aphrodisiac qualities are easily extracted and only small amounts are needed.

Turmeric root A sprinkle of this golden magic helps bring warmth to your digestion and a little more life to your life. Because turmeric helps increase the flow of blood deep into your tissues and organs, it brings more nutrition and health to your whole body and mind.

Nutmeg Believed to 'hold the energy in', nutmeg is calming and helps to break the tiring sleep-awake-sleep-awake pattern of transient insomnia.

Ashwagandha root This is one of nature's greatest gifts – it helps us sleep well, therefore giving us more energy. Its Latin name is *Withania somnifera*, alluding to its gentle soporific effects, which are accentuated when it's used at night and with milk. Ashwagandha means 'the smell of a horse' – you won't smell like a horse the next day, but you will wake with the grace, elegance and vigour of one.

Energise & Rejuvenate

This is the quintessential herbal tea: earthy, herbaceous, grassy and brimming with minerals.

Nourishing nettle tea

Nettle leaf 30g/1oz

This will serve 2–3 cups of nettle brew.

Put the nettle leaf in a pot. Add 500ml/18fl oz cold water. Leave to steep for 2–4 hours (or even overnight) and then strain for a truly nourishing brew that you can drink throughout the day.

Nettle leaf Nettle gets its name from the old Anglo-Dutch word *netel* meaning 'needle'. For those who have experienced its sharp sting, I needn't say more. Its role in human culture is laudable, notably as a fibre for making clothes, nets, paper, dye, vegetarian cheese rennet and beer – and of course, it aids our health.

It's a renowned *alterative* tonic, meaning that it increases the functioning of the body to alter and enhance health. It's often used by people needing extra nutrition, such as in pregnancy or when breastfeeding, because it contains so many nutrients including Vitamin B, C, K, beta-carotene, protein and essential fatty acids, as well as minerals (potassium, calcium, chromium, magnesium, silica, manganese, phosphorus, iron, selenium). Its astringency gives it the ability to stop bleeding, helping to balance heavy periods as well as nose bleeds.

Nettle can be both rejuvenative and detoxifying – as a rejuvenative tonic, it can build blood; as a detoxifier, it can dry wastes and clear mucus congestion. It's often used as a 'spring cleanser' and its cleansing effects extend to the urinary system (tackling cystitis), as well as the skin (for eczema and psoriasis) and joints (for arthritis.) Nettle is an all-round green-powerhouse.

Energise & Rejuvenate

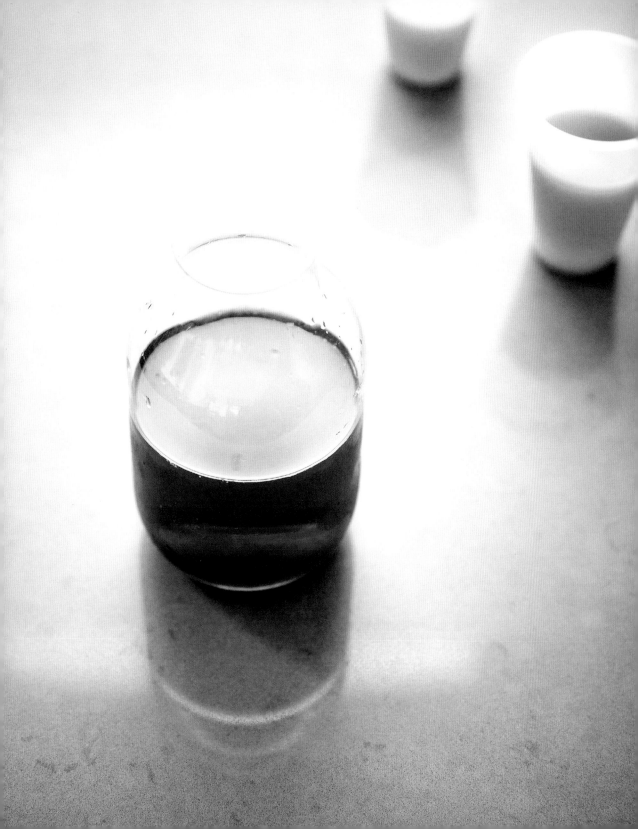

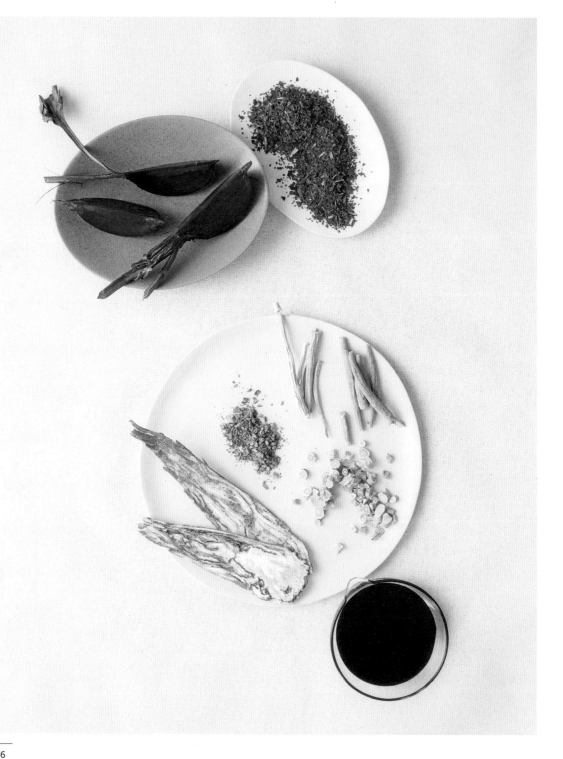

Heavenly empress vitality tonic

Blood is obviously a very special part of our bodies: it nourishes the skin, the organs, the tissues and more, and brings with it oxygen and *prana* – the ancient Indian expression for the immaterial force that animates life. This tonic syrup is a spin on an old herbal molasses recipe used for strengthening the blood. I've 'globalised' it to include herbs from Ayurveda, Chinese and European herbal traditions. It requires a bit of effort to make as it combines the principles of preparing a tea and a soup.

Nettle leaf 30g/1oz
Astragalus root 20g/¾oz
Chinese angelica root 20g/¾oz
Yellow dock root 20g/¾oz
Shatavari root 10g/⅓oz
Ashwagandha root 10g/⅓oz
Beetroot 1 fresh root
Molasses 1kg/35oz

This recipe makes about 1 month's supply. Store the liquid in a bottle in the fridge.

Take 2 tbsp 2 times per day to help build strength, nourish your blood and bring rejuvenation.

Put the nettle leaf in a pot. Add 500ml/18fl oz cold water. Leave to steep for 4 hours and then strain. Add the remaining ingredients (except the molasses) to a heavy-bottomed pan with a lid. Simmer in 750ml/26fl oz water with the lid on for 35 minutes, then strain. (You can add the strained herbs to your compost.) Mix the two strained liquids together in a pan. You should have about 1 litre/35fl oz of liquid – if you need to reduce the liquid, gently simmer in the pan with the lid off. Once you have 1 litre/35fl oz of liquid, add the molasses.

Vegetarians and pre-menopausal women especially benefit from this tonic. Even though the herbs in this formula have low levels of nutrients themselves, they have been shown to enhance iron-binding capacity and increase haemoglobin as well as B12 levels, especially when taken with molasses.

Continued overleaf

Energise & Rejuvenate

Heavenly empress vitality tonic

Nettle leaf Nature's nutrient scavenger, nettle draws nutrients from the soil and makes them accessible to us. Nettle is so mineral-rich that it actually has a minerally metallic flavour.

Astragalus root A great herb for improving energy levels, immunity and vitality. It is sweet and replenishing to your energy, lifting it and you upwards.

Chinese angelica root One of the great blood-nourishing tonics, this relative of lovage and our European angelica supports the building and creation of nature's life-giving essence.

Yellow dock root Best paired with molasses in order to nourish blood, yellow dock root's tonifying properties also have a positive effect on the liver.

Shatavari root The ultimate rejuvenative, especially for women. Shatavari helps nourish the reproductive system, which is essentially fed by our blood.

Ashwagandha root Containing a little iron, ashwagandha builds blood strength. When our blood is strong then we can be calm and grounded; if our blood is weak, we can be more emotionally vulnerable.

Beetroot Packed with iron, calcium, Vitamin A and C, beetroot is the epitome of a nutritious vegetable. Blood-red, beetroot also contains a pigment known as betanin which is a strong detoxifier for the liver and also a blood builder.

Molasses This sticky syrup is a mineral- and nutrient-rich elixir made from a by-product of sugar production that is low in sucrose and high in Vitamin B6 and minerals such as iron, calcium, magnesium, manganese and potassium. Especially rich in iron, it is an excellent blood tonic and is known to strengthen the blood, in turn helping to strengthen our spirit.

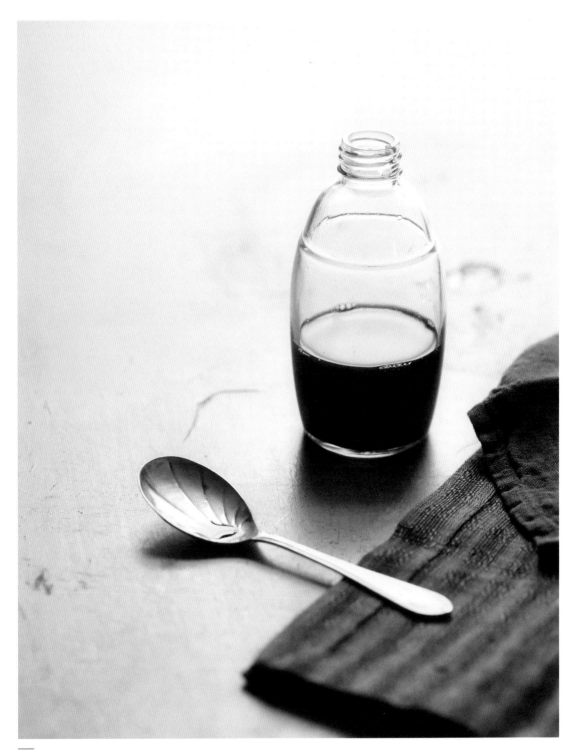

It's hard to beat a classic. Fresh, sweet and uplifting, this is a drink to enjoy freely throughout the day.

Peppermint & licorice

Peppermint leaf 6g
Licorice root 3g

This will serve 2–3 cups of a classic herbal tea.

Put all of the ingredients in a pot. Add 500ml/18fl oz freshly boiled filtered water. Leave to steep for 5–10 minutes, then strain.

Peppermint leaf Sweet, cooling, light and ascendant, peppermint balances all three constitutional types in Ayurveda. The aromatic leaf is a famous digestif that eases stomach spasms and reduces digestive discomfort. Both our mind and digestive system have the jobs of assimilating the challenges life throws at us – keep your digestion smooth, and your thinking will be too. Drinking mint tea is a good way of helping your stomach to help your mind.

Licorice root Very sweet, a little cooling and known as a *demulcent*, licorice is a herbal tea favourite. A remarkable quality of licorice is that its sweetness is 50 times greater than sucrose. In Sanskrit, Latin and Chinese the words for licorice translate as 'sweet stick' (*yastimadhu* in Sanskrit, *Glycyrrhiza* in Latin and *gan cao* in Chinese). Its sweet flavour reflects its tonifying qualities: it directly strengthens the kidneys, nourishes the nervous system, soothes upset digestion and brings peaceful energy.

Energise & Rejuvenate

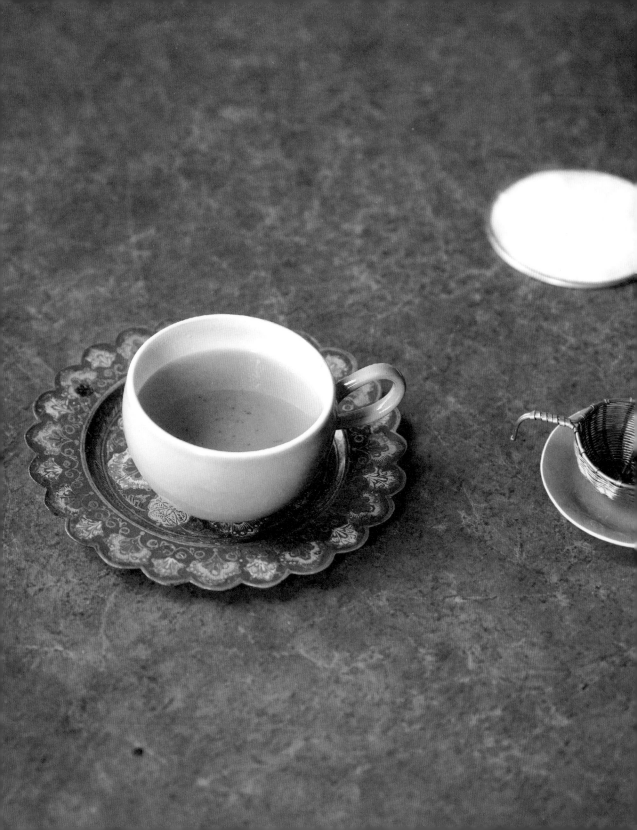

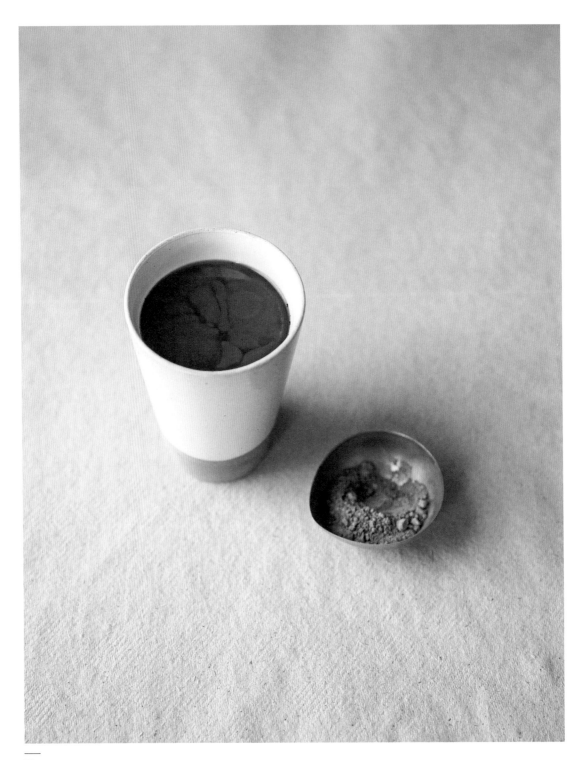

Perfect for that I-need-something-satisfying-now moment. Make this tea for some pure herbal indulgence.

Cacao orange rejuvenator

Ginseng root 3g
Roasted chicory root 5g
Orange peel 3g
Licorice root 2g
Cacao powder 1g per cup
Orange essential oil a drop per cup
Honey to taste

This will serve 2–3 cups of rich and rejuvenating tea.

Put the ginseng in a pan with a lid. Add 200ml/7fl oz cold water and simmer with the lid on for 30 minutes. Add the roasted chicory root, orange peel and licorice root to the pan along with 400ml/14fl oz freshly boiled filtered water. Leave to steep for 10–15 minutes. Meanwhile, prepare the cups by adding cacao powder to each one. Once the tea has steeped, strain and pour it onto the cacao powder in the cups. Whisk and finish with a drop of orange essential oil in each cup. (If you're short on time, skip simmering the ginseng, or leave it out.)

Ginseng root Very precious (it takes years to grow!), ginseng root is ideally boiled to extract the best value out of it. It is one of nature's finest energy boosters, immediately lifting your vitality upwards, helping you feel ready to move.
Roasted chicory root A favourite bitter tonic. Roasting chicory brings out the flavour and when used in tea it makes for a dark, rich drink. You can replace this with roasted dandelion too.
Orange peel This tastes like vitality itself. Orange peel assists digestion and clears a muzzy head.
Licorice root Licorice is a wonder rejuvenator for adrenal and nervous systems. It helps you manage stress and to tolerate it better.
Cacao powder Beautifully indulgent, cacao is a mood lifter, aphrodisiac and nourishing tonic all in one.

For the best all-round effect, use organic whole root ginseng slices and not just the tails. See Herb Suppliers on p232 for good sources.

Sold at chai stalls all over India, this is the Indian take on a British classic: a warming black tea gently spiced and sweetened. The saviour of many low blood sugar moments, it is rich, sweet, spicy and energising, and ideally enjoyed as a treat on a cold winter's day. As well as tasting fantastic, the cardamom and ginger warm digestion and help counteract any mucus the milk might produce. It's best made with the strongest tea you can find – Assam is a favourite.

Maharajah's majestic chai

Assam black tea loose leaf
  (or rip a teabag open) 3g
Fresh ginger root 2 slices
Cardamom pod 3 pods
Milk (any type) 200ml/7fl oz
Sugar a pinch per glass (optional)

Serves 4 piping hot chais when served in authentic chai glasses.

Simmer 200ml/7fl oz water in a saucepan and as it comes to a rolling boil add the black tea. Add the fresh ginger slices and the cardamom pods. Simmer for a couple of minutes, then add the milk. Just as this starts to boil sprinkle in the sugar (if using), then take off the heat. Strain immediately, and serve. Blow to cool and sip with friends.

Ginger root Ginger is often used in chai for its warming and digestive-enhancing qualities.
Cardamom pod This green globe of tropical treasure helps the chai to taste delightful and, like any good cup of chai, it helps to awaken your mind. It also helps to reduce the mucus-forming effects of drinking milk.

Energise & Rejuvenate

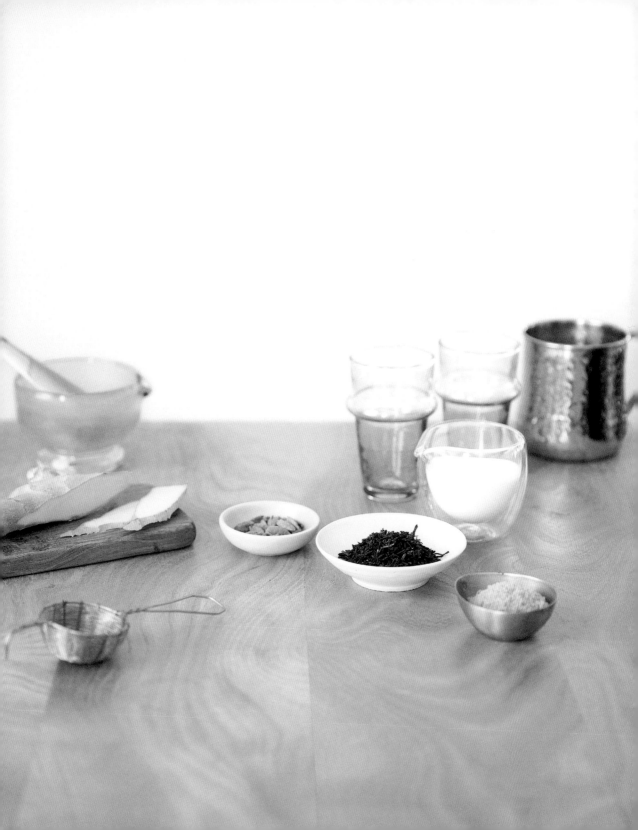

A caffeine-free alternative to Maharajah's Majestic Chai (p84).
I drink this whenever I fancy a warming taste of the tropics.

Sweet herb chai

Cinnamon bark 3g
Ginger root powder 2g
Cardamom pod 2g
Licorice root 2g
Vanilla pod 1g (or to taste)

This will serve 2–3 cups of tropical vitality.

Put all of the ingredients in a pot or pan with a lid. Add 500ml/18fl oz freshly boiled filtered water. Leave to steep for 10–15 minutes (or for a stronger chai simmer in the pan with the lid on for 10–15 minutes), then strain.

Cinnamon bark Spicy-sweet cinnamon bark warms you up and gets you going.
Ginger root Warm ginger is an essential ingredient in every chai. Great for digestion and giving you a little tickle, helping to perk you up.
Cardamom pod This fragrant pod awakens your mind and makes the chai an authentic one.
Licorice root Licorice is a fantastic sweetener and a lot healthier than sugar.
Vanilla pod The delight of the tropics, vanilla brings pleasure to mind, body, soul and tastebuds alike.

Energise & Rejuvenate

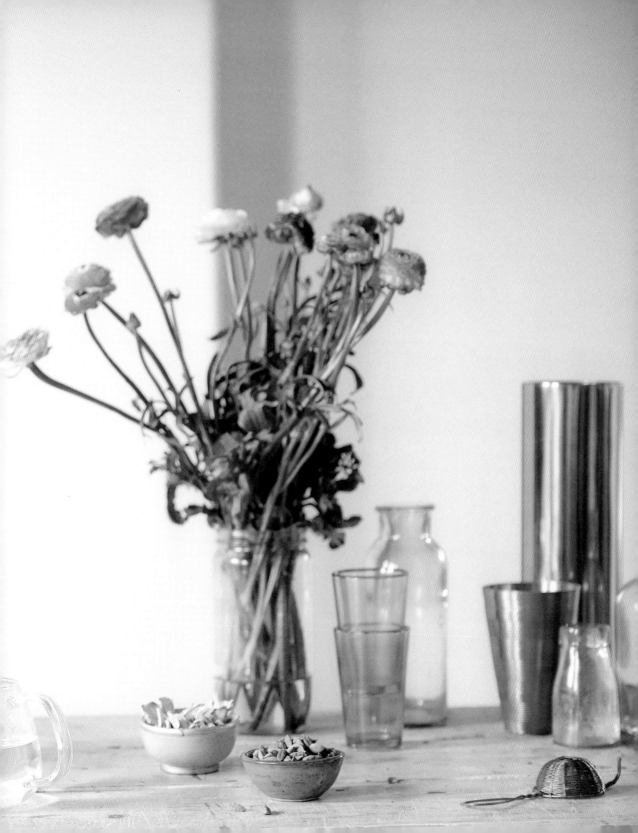

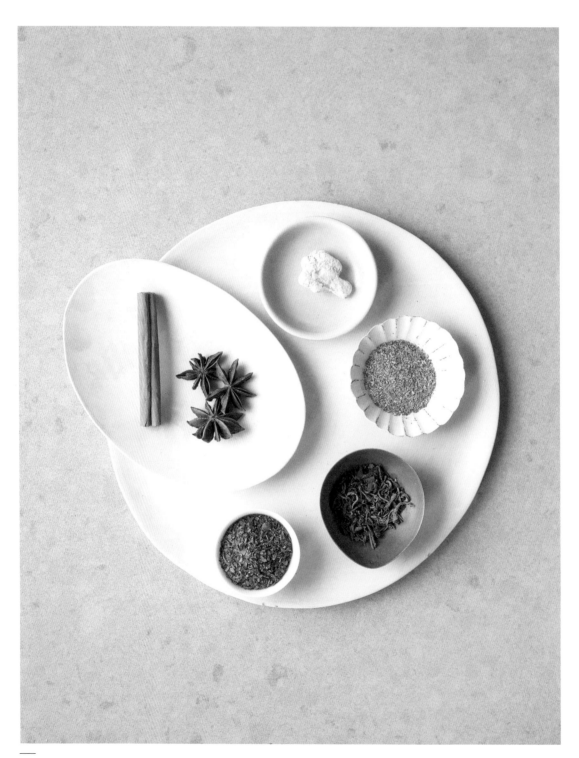

Rise like a star

This is an energising tea to get you going in the morning or when you need a little boost. The fragrant spices provide herbal oomph, making this a great tea for sluggish mornings.

Star anise 3g
Cinnamon bark 2g
Spearmint leaf 2g
Green tea 1g
Ginger root powder 1g
Licorice root 1g

This will serve 2–3 cups of lethargy-banishing tea.

Put all of the ingredients in a pot. Add 500ml/18fl oz freshly boiled filtered water. Leave to steep for 10–15 minutes, then strain.

Star anise This celestial-looking spice is wonderfully aromatic and has a unique sweet aniseed flavour. It awakens your senses and reminds you how delicious life can be.

Cinnamon bark A favourite of early explorers seeking its therapeutic benefits, this fragrant bark warms digestion and increases circulation. It is very good for clearing a stuffy feeling in the chest after the torpor of the night.

Spearmint leaf Mildly warming to digestion, spearmint helps to clear any heaviness or listlessness and helps to lift your spirits.

Green tea Green tea contains small amounts of caffeine that can help stimulate. It is also mildly bitter and astringent, helping to rid any feelings of lethargy.

Ginger root This spicy wonder root is great for balancing heavy *kapha* feelings and is a real energiser.

Licorice root An active adrenal tonic, licorice's sweet root nourishes your energy levels.

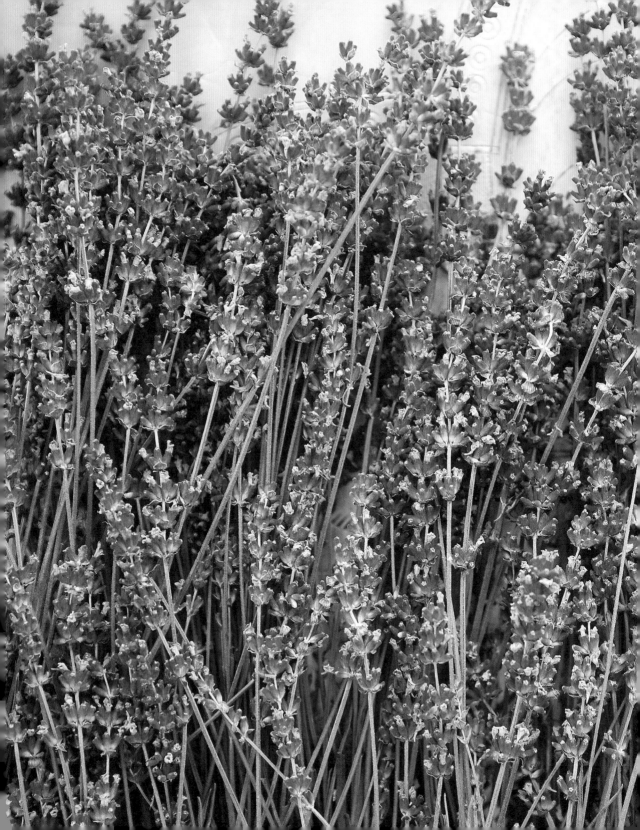

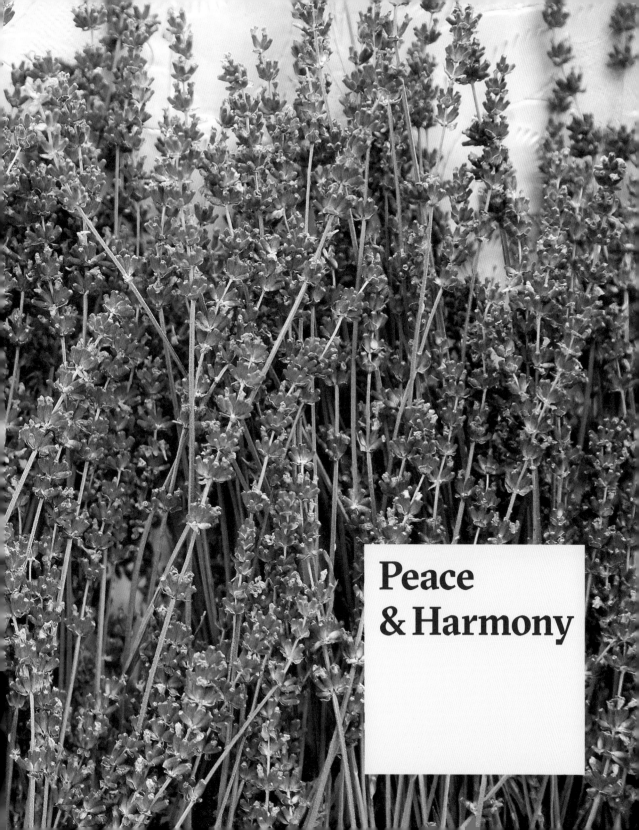

Peace
& Harmony

"Within you there is a stillness and a sanctuary to which you can retreat at any time and be yourself."

Hermann Hesse

This thought-provoking quote by novelist, poet and literary mystic Hermann Hesse reminds me that, although it doesn't always feel like it, I am in charge of my world and am always afforded the opportunity of finding some peace inside of myself.

In a way, we all live under stress, and that's not necessarily a bad thing. Gravity is a grounding stress that keeps us on Earth; and the pull of the sun's gravitational stress holds the Earth in an ellipse so perfectly placed that life on our planet can flourish. However too much stress can push any object – or person – to the limit.

Stress is implicated in many health problems from insomnia and dermatitis to IBS and overt anxiety. Ayurveda perceives the symptoms of stress as 'living beyond our threshold' or 'living beyond our means'. If you are living with a stress overdraft, then it makes sense to recredit our reserves of peace and harmony so that we can better process the stresses we face.

There are lots of ways we can manage our daily challenges, including simple breathing exercises, meditation, a soothing massage, or using a spectrum of healing plants that can sedate, stimulate, nourish, feed and relax the nervous system.

Here are some of nature's herbal offerings that can bring a sense of peace, space, calm and harmony into your life. I would recommend drinking them regularly.

For gram to teaspoon conversion see p24

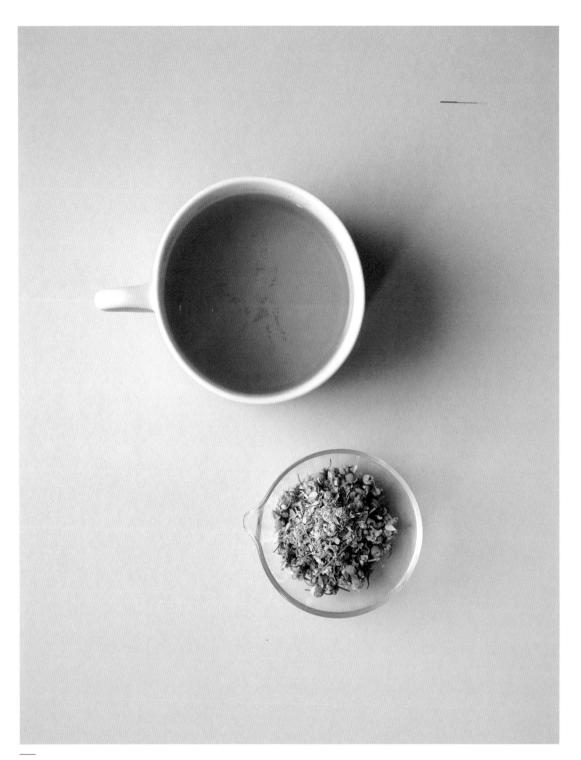

Chamomile's exquisite yellow flowers are full of a delicate sweetness that helps to soothe the soul. Just smelling them makes you feel more you.

Cool chamomile

Chamomile flower 6g

This will serve 2–3 cups of smooth chamomile tea.

Put the chamomile flowers in a pot. Add 500ml/18fl oz freshly boiled filtered water. Leave to steep for 10–15 minutes, then strain.

Don't confuse chamomile with Roman chamomile (*Anthemis nobilis*), which although is full of benefits, is much more bitter and not a very pleasant drink.

If you have sore eyes you can use a chamomile teabag (after you have enjoyed the cup of tea and it's cooled down) to place over them. Alternatively, soak a flannel in a little of this tea and squeeze. Then lie back, put the cooled flannel over your eyes and relax for a few minutes.

Chamomile flower A very delicate flower that stores the majority of its precious essential oil in the pollen – the yellow parts of the flower head. Chamomile's essential oil is a complex combination of many individual oils that turns blue when it is distilled into a pure essential oil. As well as having a wonderful aroma, the oil has anti-inflammatory, antispasmodic and antimicrobial properties.

Most mass-produced chamomile teas are made with lots of stems, so they don't have very high levels of these important compounds, or a very good flavour. So try to use chamomile pollen (as Pukka does in the Three Chamomile tea) or the whole flower so that you get the best benefit and flavour.

Chamomile's fresh, grassy and herbaceous flavours join sweet and mildly bitter notes, which help to cool and lighten your whole being. It is a popular herb for relaxing the nervous system and is often used to induce good sleep, settle restless legs and calm digestive, muscular and uterine spasms. Its ability to balance hormone levels such as oestrogen, as well as stop spasmodic pain (such as period pain), make it a valuable herb for supporting women's health. These benefits to women's health are reflected in chamomile's botanical name, *Matricaria recutita*, derived from the Latin word *matrix*, meaning 'womb'.

You can always rely on chamomile to help with mild *vata* anxiety and offer you a protective barrier from stress and strife. It's a good herb for children too, as it soothes teething, tummy upsets and restless nights.

Chamomile's mild bitter flavour makes it a wonderful digestif, helping to ease indigestion, bloating, griping cramps and gastritis as well as protecting from ulcers and acidic *pitta* inflammation. When your body is relaxed so is your mind – tune into your 'gut' feeling and turn to chamomile if you find yourself in a moment of distress.

A cup of love

A blend of flowers bringing you some of nature's finest love. Drink to soothe a broken heart or feed you when you just want a sip of love.

Chamomile flower 3g
Limeflower 2g
Marigold (calendula) petal 2g
Rose flower 1g
Lavender flower 1g
Licorice root 1g

This will serve 3 cups of love.

Put all of the ingredients in a pot. Add 500ml/18fl oz freshly boiled filtered water. Leave to steep for 10–15 minutes, then strain and let the love flow.

Chamomile flower This little yellow flower brings peace to your heart. By relaxing your body it relaxes your mind and helps you get in touch with your feelings.

Limeflower The heavenly flowers of this enormous tree relax you into a blissful state where you are ready to connect with love.

Marigold petal The mother of all healing plants. Also known as calendula (because it often flowers for a full calendar year), it brings joy and colour to your tea and to your life. Marigold is a renowned healer of all types of trauma, both physical and emotional. It's a specific for skin irritation, and you can use a pure marigold tea as a compress on burns and sores. Its ability to bring balance is especially useful when a menstrual cycle is irregular or painful.

Rose flower The ultimate aroma of *amore*. Rose has a special affinity with the heart, helping you to open up to the unlimited possibilities of love.

Lavender flower Just smelling lavender cheers your heart, soothes pain and makes you feel like anything is possible.

Licorice root Sweet and calming, licorice is used to enhance feelings of love and compassion, as well as offset some of the slightly tangy notes in this floral tea.

This tea makes a great foot-soak to help you relax and bask in the waters of love. It actually looks amazing with all the petals in. Just scale up the measures for the tea above and soak your feet in the warm water for some deep herbal bliss.

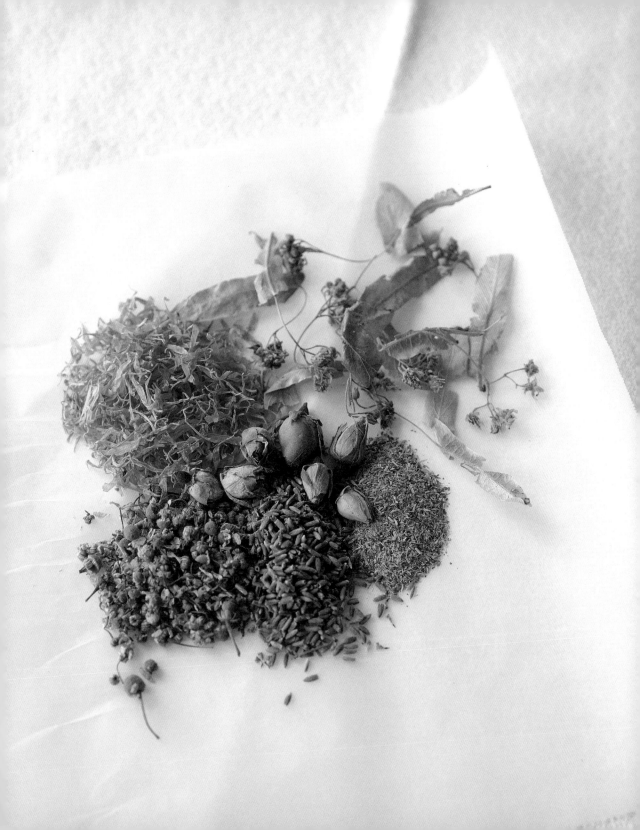

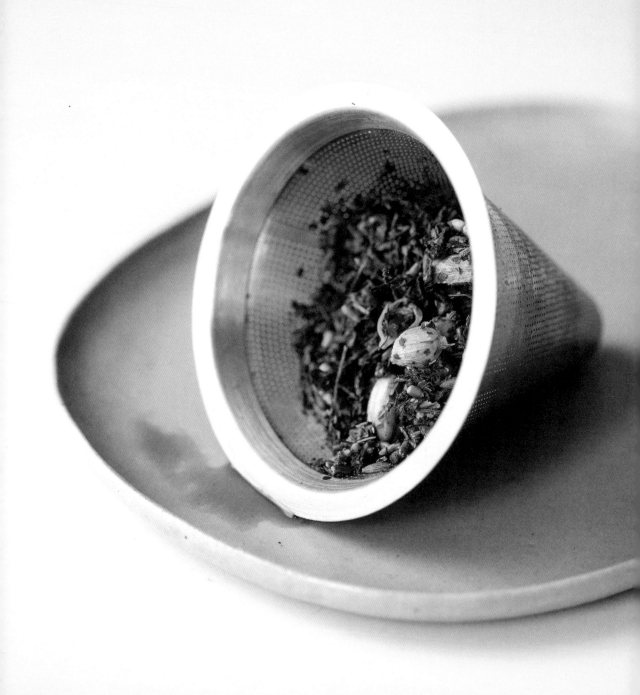

Pure clarity

This tea brings you one step closer to enlightenment. It turns a lightbulb on in your head so that you can think straight in the face of life's unrelenting challenges. Use it when you need better concentration, clearer thinking and a sharper memory.

Tulsi leaf 3g
Rosemary leaf 2g
Cardamom pod 2g
Spearmint leaf 2g
Lavender flower 1g

This will serve 2 cups of enlightenment.

Put all of the ingredients in a pot.
Add 500ml/18fl oz freshly boiled filtered water. Leave to steep for 10–15 minutes, then strain.

Tulsi leaf Deeply rooted in Indian culture, this revered leaf is also known as holy basil. It gently improves our response to physical and mental challenges. Tulsi is rich in antioxidants and famed for its protective anti-ageing properties. In Ayurveda it is renowned for increasing *prana*, which uplifts your spirits and paves the way towards deeper clarity.

Rosemary leaf Remember, rosemary is for remembrance. Full of rejuvenative wonder, it's a powerful brain tonic that quickly makes you feel more alert.

Cardamom pod Strongly uplifting, cardamom banishes that muzzy-head foggy feeling.

Spearmint leaf A touch of spearmint lifts all the herbs to your head – it contains essential oils that move upwards, helping to keep your brain as bright as a lightbulb.

Lavender flower A favourite for a heavy head, lavender helps you to relax so you can think more clearly.

Peace & Harmony

Peace tea

These herbs help you move closer to peace, one sip at a time.

Chamomile flower 3g
Spearmint leaf 2g
Lavender flower 2g
Licorice root 1g
Cannabis leaf 1g (optional, use hops as a replacement)
Olive leaf 1g (optional)

This will serve 2–3 cups of stillness.

Put all of the ingredients in a pot. Add 500ml/18fl oz freshly boiled filtered water. Leave to steep for 10–15 minutes, then strain and breathe in.

Chamomile flower If you know chamomile you know peace. It takes you to a place of stillness from where you can find tranquility.

Spearmint leaf This lightening leaf is fresh and cleansing, helping you feel comfortable with who and how you are. Its essential oils are known to help relax your nervous system and bring tranquility when you need it most.

Lavender flower Gently wafting clouds of fragrant peace, lavender dips you into a purple pool of calm.

Licorice root Beloved by Buddhists for enhancing clarity during meditation, this sweet tonic root supports, nourishes and balances the entire system. Renowned in Ayurveda for strengthening the nervous system and the intellectual quality of your brain, licorice actually rejuvenates your mind.

Cannabis leaf This is optional and only suggested for people living in countries where it's legal to procure. Some of the resinous compounds help relax your nervous system and give the tea a deeply herbal taste.

Hops An alternative replacement to cannabis leaf, hops are a member of the *Cannabinacea* family, and as any beer drinker knows, have a gentle mellowing effect.

Olive leaf Carried by doves as a peace offering, olive leaf doesn't taste that interesting, but its potent antioxidants are a welcome offering for stressed-out cells. Add it as a symbolic offering on your path to peace.

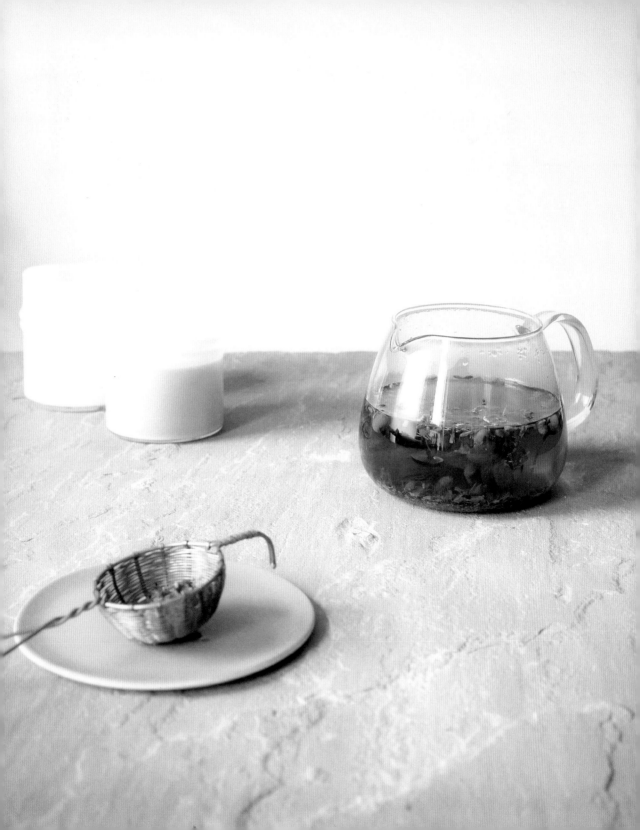

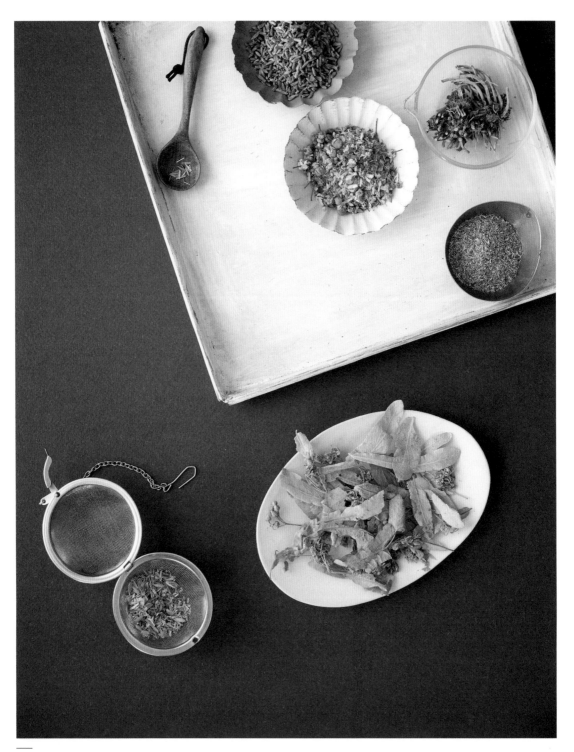

A blissfully restful tea that is sweet and soothing. Helpful for anyone who doesn't fall to sleep easily or wakes in the night. Let the herbs sweeten your dreams.

Sweet dreams

Oat straw flowering top 3g
Limeflower 2g
Chamomile flower 2g
Lavender flower 1g
Valerian root 1g
Licorice root 1g

This will serve 2–3 cups of sweet dreams.

Put all of the ingredients in a pot.
Add 500ml/18fl oz freshly boiled filtered water. Leave to steep for 10–15 minutes, then strain, sip and fall to sleep.

Oat straw flowering top This sweet herb calms you from your head right to your toes. Picked just as they are flowering, oat straw tops feed your nervous system and help it move into a relaxed mode. (Harvested before the oat grain kernel forms, they are gluten free too.)

Limeflower A sweet and delicate herb that helps calm the nervous system and brings restful sleep. It makes the tea sweet and silky.

Chamomile flower Everyone's favourite nighttime herb to help promote a soft sweet sleep.

Lavender flower Beautiful purple flowers that soothe your heart, mind and senses.

Valerian root The renowned sleep-inducing root is aromatic, grounding and calming. Some people hate the smell and some people love it – either way, it's quite pungent so only use a little.

Licorice root Grounding licorice helps to calm your mind as you drift off into dream land.

Take it easy

As stress first aggravates the nervous system and then the digestion, this is a tea designed to tackle the problem in reverse. It first relaxes the digestive system and then calms you down. It is Pukka's original *vata*-stress balancing tea.

Fennel seed 3g
Chamomile flower 3g
Cardamom pod 2g
Ginger root powder 2g
Marshmallow root 2g
Oat straw flowering top 2g
Licorice root 1g

This will serve 2 cups of calm.

Put all of the ingredients in a pot. Add 500ml/18fl oz freshly boiled filtered water. Leave to steep for 10–15 minutes, then strain and let it all hang out.

Fennel seed Fennel seed is a marvellous herb for aiding digestion. People prone to nervousness and anxiety easily get upset digestion and fennel can help to counteract this. Its high essential oil content works to relax and soothe muscles in the digestive system. It helps to prevent cramps and gripes by reducing wind and bloating.

Chamomile flower When we are stressed the nervous system is taxed. This world famous yellow flower calms the nervous system, while its rich mineral content feeds the whole system. It is also a renowned digestion-relaxing herb that alleviates cramps and spasms.

Cardamom pod This tasty tropical seed is wonderfully aromatic. It helps the digestion to function efficiently. It is also warming and helps to relax any tightness in the abdomen.

Ginger root This spicy root encourages the digestive system to function perfectly. It stimulates digestive enzymes and maximises our ability to absorb the nutrients in food.

Marshmallow root This root is very soft and healing for all the mucous membranes of the body. It specifically counteracts dryness in the membranes and inflammation in your digestion, lungs and urinary and reproductive systems.

Oat straw flowering top Sweet and soothing oat straw nourishes and calms the nervous system.

Licorice root This sweet root is great for easing spasms and inflammation in the digestive tract. It is also excellent at strengthening weakness in the body, especially when caused by stress and anxiety.

Peace & Harmony

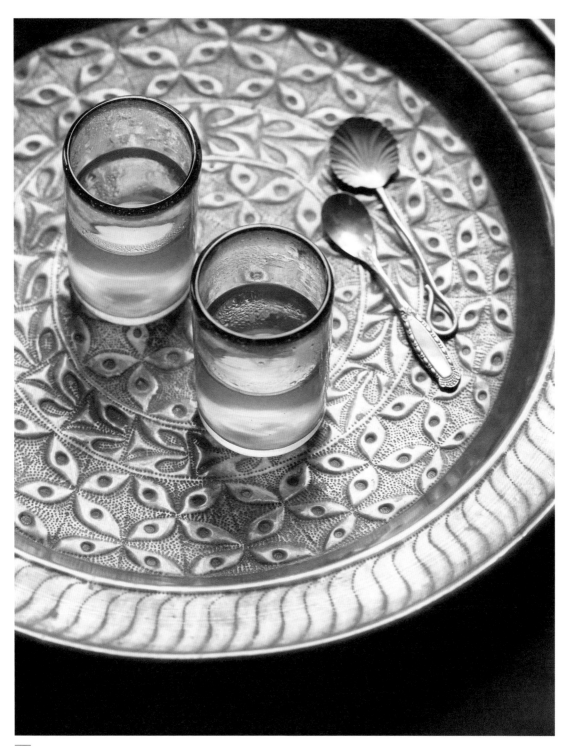

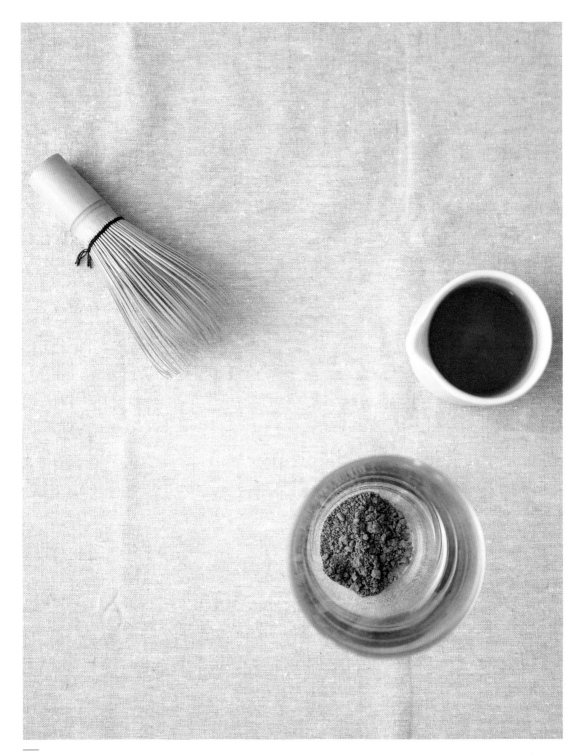

A good green tea is transcendental, taking you to your inner Shangri-La. There are so many delicious green leaf teas such as Sencha, Long Jing, Gyokuro, Gunpowder, Dragonwell and Green Cloud – simply choose one you like. I prefer them when they are whole leaf with a bright greenness.

Green matcha zen

Green tea 4g
Matcha 1g per cup

This will serve 2 cups of what many consider to be a taste and experience of Nirvana.

Put the green tea in a warmed pot. Add 500ml/18fl oz freshly boiled filtered water left off the boil for a minute or two (green tea is best made with water around 80–85°C/175–185°F in order to retain its sweet and astringent flavour). Leave to steep for 3–5 minutes, then strain. Meanwhile, add the matcha powder to each cup. Once the green tea is steeped, pour over the matcha, whisk and serve. If you are using a good green tea, you will be able to refill the teapot for a second cup.

Green tea Green tea is made from the unfermented leaves of *Camellia sinensis*, otherwise known as the tea plant. After water, it's the most popular drink in the world. It tastes sweet, delicately bitter and astringent, and feels light and dry. Bubbling with some of nature's finest protective antioxidant polyphenols, green tea is lauded as a valuable part of our daily diet. Paradoxically, it helps to both calm and energise. It's good for digestion, protects the liver and supports clarity of mind. One of the reasons we love it so much is that it helps us feel bright, present and in the moment.

Matcha Ceremonial matcha is made from the young top buds of shaded tea bushes. The tea bushes are shaded for a couple of days before harvesting to increase the amount of amino acids, which makes the tea sweeter. After harvest, the leaves are ground to the finest powder in stone mills. A very important factor is the temperature the matcha is subjected to, so the milling is extremely slow in order to avoid high temperatures that can destroy its quality. The fibre is extracted from the powdered tea, which enhances the polyphenol content and the smooth, rich flavour.

Growing the matcha under shade increases the volume of healing chlorophyll as well as the L-Theanine, amino acids and polyphenols such as EGCG (epigallocatechin gallate). These natural compounds add to the sweet and savoury mineral flavour, known as umami. The rare amino acid L-Theanine helps to nourish neurotransmitters in the brain, which have a positive influence on our mood and sense of inner peace. L-Theanine works synergistically with the low levels of caffeine in green tea, and matcha helps to bring a deep sense of calm as well as alertness. In fact, L-Theanine helps release alpha-waves in the brain, which are also produced after a deep meditation. L-Theanine is five times higher in matcha than green tea.

Peace & Harmony

Oolong

Oolong is a favourite of tea connoisseurs. It's made from light semi-fermented green clusters of leaves with flavours ranging from creamy to honeyed to citrus. I prefer the lighter style of greeny-blueish floral oolongs, but the darker more malty Chinese varieties are also popular. With names like Ti Kuan Yin, meaning the Goddess of Compassion, and Iron Buddha, drinking oolong teas can be as inspiring as their names.

Oolong 3g

This will serve 1 cup of inspiring tea.

Put the oolong in a pot or cup. Add 250ml/9fl oz freshly boiled filtered water left off the boil for a minute or two (oolong leaves are tightly wrapped and unfurl best in water that's around 85–90°C/ 185–195°F, which helps them to retain their sweet flavour). Leave to steep for about 3 minutes before tasting. Enjoy the first cup and then you can top up a couple more times for further delight – oolong just keeps getting better.

Oolong Oolong teas make your life better and longer. They are renowned for managing weight as their antioxidant polyphenols help to enhance your metabolism and reduce fat levels. They regulate blood sugar and insulin levels, which helps you avoid sugar highs and lows. This prevents excess blood sugar from being converted to fat, so you could say the side-effect of drinking oolong is that it balances your weight. Another gift from the Goddess of Compassion is making your skin glow, which in essence makes you as beautiful as a Buddha.

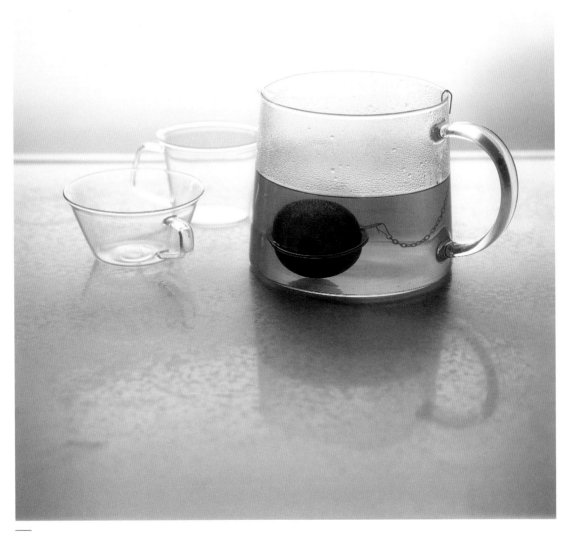

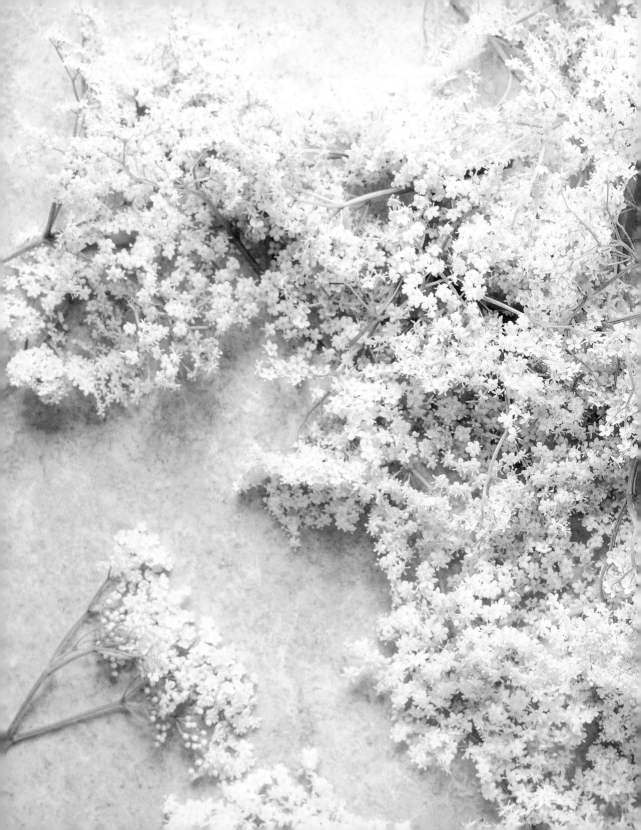

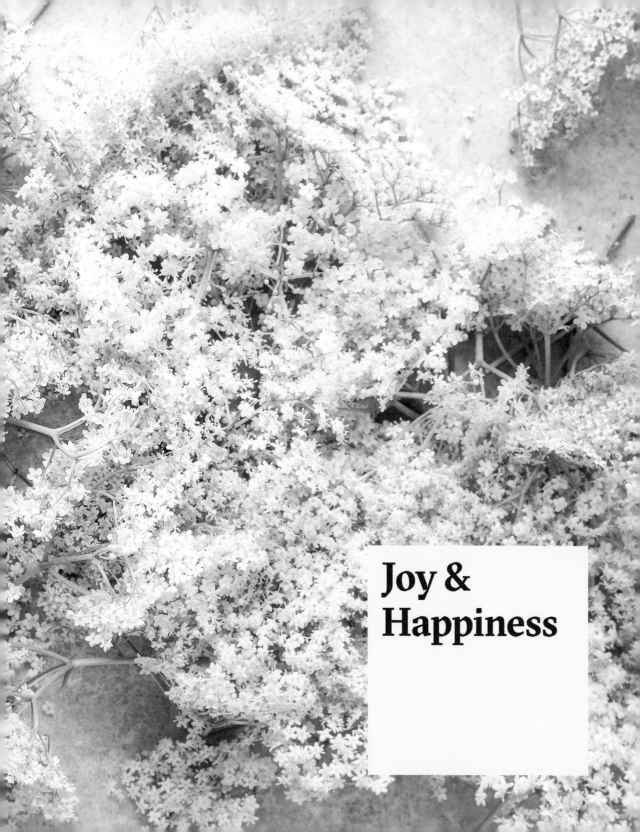

Joy &
Happiness

"May all beings be happy. May they live in safety and joy."
The Buddha's words on kindness from the Metta Sutta

We all need a little pick-me-up from time to time. Life can be challenging and demand a lot from us. When it asks for more than we can handle, it can get us down, causing us to lose our natural sparkle. If that happens too often, then we can end up walking around without no sparkle at all – and that's a problem that we need to solve.

One of the best ways to bring a bit of brightness into our day is to spend some time remembering and appreciating what we have. Sitting for a few moments in gratitude and noting the things and people we love in our lives can bring a fresh perspective and remind us how full our glass really is. This might be as simple as appreciating feeling warm, or having a soft bed. Or it can be a feeling of gratitude for life itself.

Life offers us the incredible potential to experience happiness. Throughout history, to a greater or lesser degree, we have relentlessly pursued happiness through relationships, religion, money, food or drugs. Of course, plants have been at the centre of this pursuit, with many being worshipped in different cultures for the transcendence and ecstasy they bring. Here are some of my favourites – these can help us step into the river of joy that perpetually runs through (or at least near to) our lives.

For gram to teaspoon conversion see p24

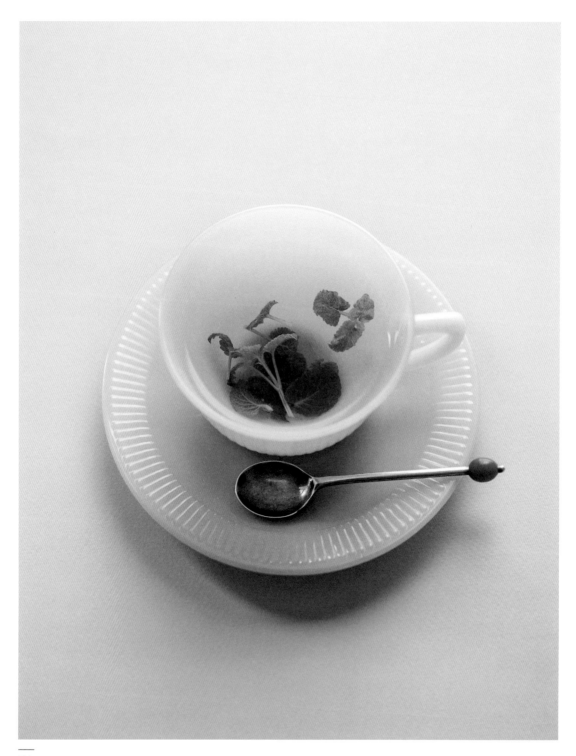

Melissa is the old name for lemon balm. It is beloved by bees and is also known as bee balm for stings. Enjoy a fresh sprig whenever you want to relax your brow and raise your spirits.

Melissa's magic

**Fresh lemon balm leaf 2 sprigs
    (the top 8cm/3¼in with 4–6 leaves)**

This will serve 1 cup of magical tea.

Put the lemon balm in a cup. Add 250ml/9fl oz freshly boiled filtered water. Leave to steep for a few minutes and enjoy with the leaves still in your cup.

Pick fresh lemon balm before it flowers for the sweetest cup. If you don't have access to any fresh lemon balm then use 1 tsp of good quality dry leaf.

If you have a lemon balm plant, pick the fresh leaves in spring and early summer and dry them gently to store for the winter.

Lemon balm leaf Its delicate lemony essential oils, as well as potent antioxidant properties, add to its ability to awaken your consciousness. Lemon balm leaf can be used as a gentle calming *carminative* herb for children and adults alike. It is a favourite for raising your mood when confronted with feelings of insecurity, anxiety and self-judgement. And it has an affinity with the thyroid and can be very beneficial for calming hyperactive people (though it is best only used occasionally for those on thyroid medication).

Overflowing with cooling properties, it helps to keep you calm and collected. Its ability to lighten tension also helps to open the mind and improve clear thinking. This 'head-opening' effect can help to ease headaches as well as blow away a low mood. It is as close to a cup of spirit-raising tea as you can get.

Let there be joy

When the chips are down and the blues have clouded your day, drink this blend of instant-happiness-herbs. Not all of life's experiences are easy, but this tea will help you digest them.

Lemon balm 3g
Limeflower 3g
Lavender flower 2g
Rosemary leaf 1g
St John's wort flowering top 1g
Rose water 1 tsp per cup
Honey a dash per cup

This will serve 2 cups of happiness.

Put all of the ingredients in a pot (except for the rose water and honey). Add 500ml/ 18fl oz freshly boiled filtered water. Leave to steep for 10–15 minutes, then strain. Add the rose water and honey to taste, then sip for joy.

Lemon balm The personification of a spirit-raising herb, lemon balm opens your mind so you can connect with your heart.
Limeflower While the sweet smell of this delicate flower brings instant happiness, the honey-like taste can also bring joy into your day.
Lavender flower Pairing beautifully with lemon balm, lavender banishes anxiety and brings joy. Just smelling lavender helps us feel better.
Rosemary leaf Happiness is all around, we just need to find it. Rosemary clears the cobwebs that can envelop our mood, making us feel alert and susceptible to an excess of jubilation.
St John's wort flowering top St John's wort is really good at helping to heal emotional wounds and move 'stuck' emotions. As the block clears, we can start to feel ourselves again.
Rose water I am in love with rose water. It does something very special inside you. Try it and see.
Honey Honey really is unique. It directs this formula to your head and brings immediate energy to your brain. St John's wort is a bit astringent, so this tea needs a sweet lubricant like honey.

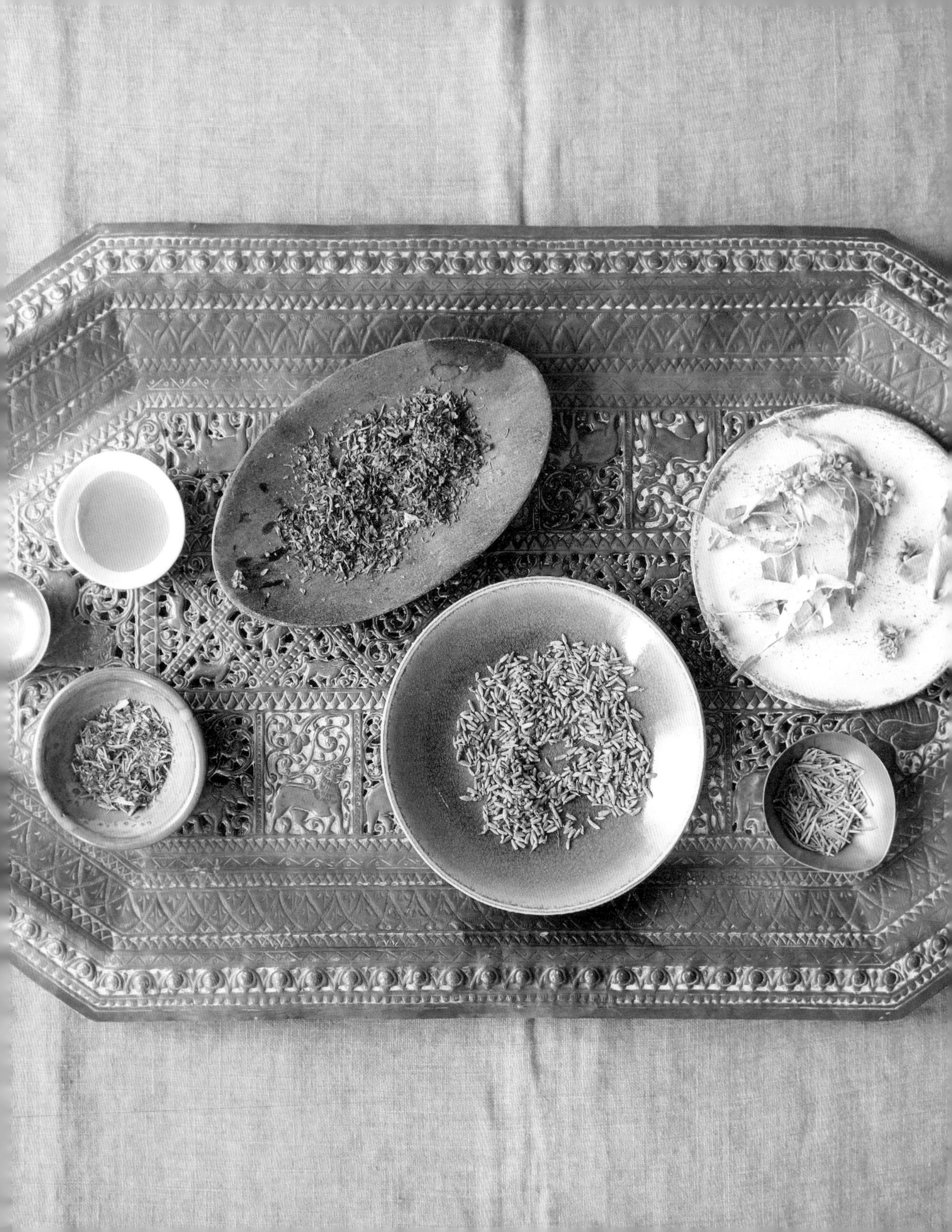

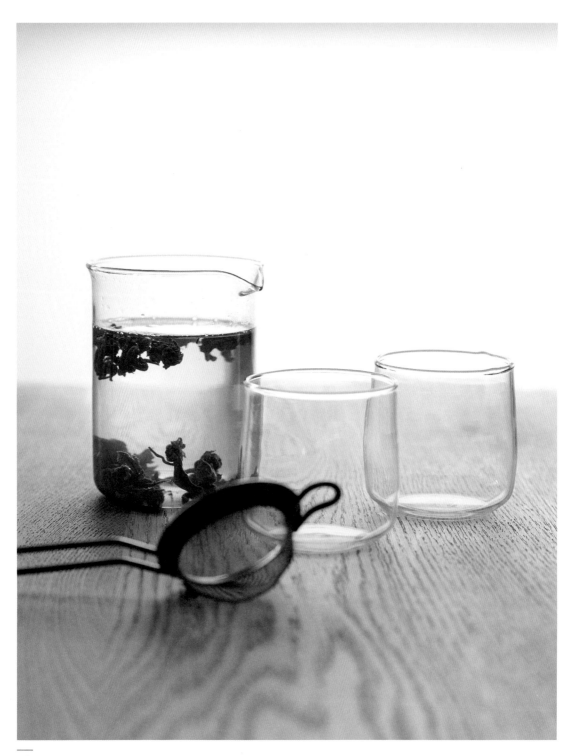

Jasmine green tea

Life would be one amazing tea short if it wasn't for jasmine. The best jasmine tea is made with high quality dry green tea leaves that are then 'steeped' overnight in fresh jasmine flowers. The more jasmine flowers the green tea is steeped in, the more delightful the tea. Look out for 'pearls' of jasmine green tea that are hand-rolled and unfurl enticingly before your eyes when you add hot water.

Jasmine green tea 2g

This will serve 1 cup of exquisite tea.

Put the jasmine green tea in a pot or cup. Add 250ml/9fl oz freshly boiled filtered water left off the boil for a minute or two (green tea is best made with water around 80–85°C/ 175–185°F in order to retain its sweet and astringent flavour). Leave to steep for about 3 minutes before tasting. Enjoy the first cup and then you can top up a couple more times for further delight.

Jasmine green tea Green tea contains all sorts of mood-lifting compounds. The caffeine energises and awakens your brain, while its amino acid L-Theanine keeps you cool as a cucumber.

Jasmine flowers immediately awaken feelings of comfort and bliss. The subtle lightness helps to raise one's consciousness to greater levels of awareness. Its sweet exotic fragrance opens the heart and gets you ready for a taste of pure joy.

Joy & Happiness

Lemon heaven

Lemon is a spritz of happiness. Its bouncy citrus can transport you to your inner heaven. The herbs in this lemon treat are light, ascendant and dispersing, bringing clarity, energy and liberation.

Fresh lemon verbena 10 leaves
Fresh lemon balm leaf 4 sprigs
Fresh lemongrass 1 stalk (or some
  leaves)
Lemon juice a twist per cup

This will serve 2 cups of the promised land.

Put all of the ingredients in a pot (except for the lemon juice). Add 500ml/18fl oz freshly boiled filtered water. Leave to steep for 10–15 minutes, then strain. Add the twist of lemon juice to each cup.

Lemon juice Lemon has a classic sour flavour, which is stimulating. Just suck on a lemon and you will see. If your digestion is sluggish it can be close to hell, if your liver is overloaded then you can behave like the devil, and if your mind is foggy it's best to go back to bed. But never fear as Lemon Heaven is here: it stimulates your digestion, squeezes your liver and awakens your mind. Brimming with a broad range of essential oils such as limone and bergamotene – also found in the bergamot oil – lemon is a sour stimulant to your digestion, immediately waking up your taste buds and your tummy.

Lemon verbena A light and delicate leaf with a light and delicate flavour. It will help to lift your mood.

Lemon balm leaf A lemony mood-lifter par excellence. It's called lemon balm for a good reason, as it can soothe a jangled digestion and a frazzled mood in no time.

Lemongrass Perhaps the spiciest of the lemony herbs in this tea, lemongrass is quite dispersing and helps to quickly move any stagnation in your digestion or mood.

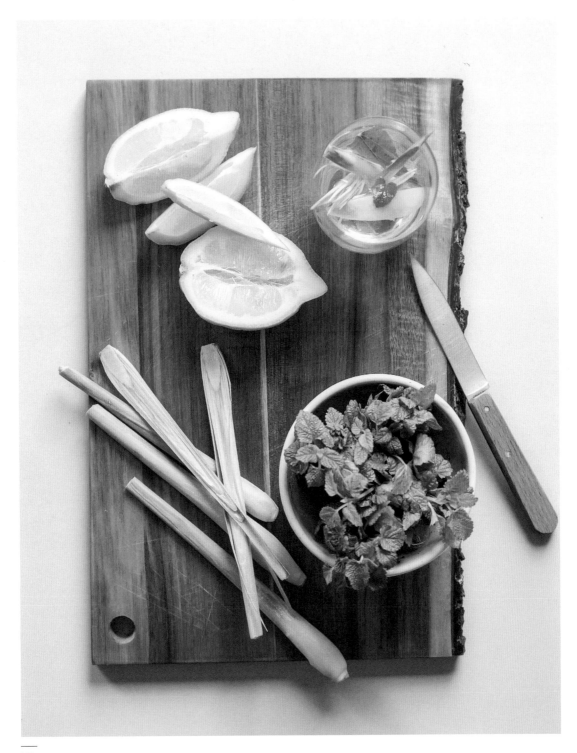

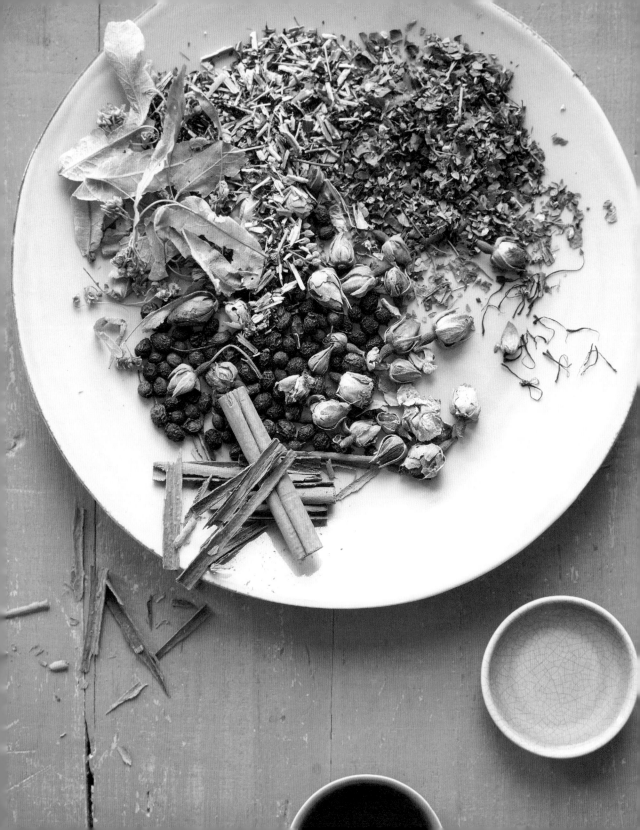

Our heart is a miracle. Not just because of its perpetual pumping, but also because it's the seat of our consciousness, directly responding to how we feel. Just as we now know that the heart has receptors responding to hormones and neuropeptides, we also know that if extreme feelings, such as anger or grief, linger for too long then they can affect the heart. Anger is a high risk factor for heart-disease just as junk food is. This is a therapeutic tea for nourishing your heart, both the physical and emotional.

Brave heart

Hawthorn berry 4g
Hawthorn leaf and flower 2g
Limeflower 2g
Cinnamon bark 2g
Motherwort 1g
Saffron 5 strands
Rose flower 1g
Pomegranate juice a glug
  (or 1 tbsp) per cup

This will serve 2 cups of a very heart-loving tea.

Put all of the ingredients in a pot (except for the pomegranate juice). Add 500ml/18fl oz freshly boiled filtered water. Leave to steep for 10–15 minutes, then strain. Add a glug of pomegranate juice to each cup.

Hawthorn berry, leaf and flower If colour is anything to go by, this vibrant red berry is one for your heart. The leaf is considered to be a specific restorative to the heart muscle, and the flower has a long history of use in aiding heart weakness. Hawthorn is my go-to herb for anyone with a broken heart or anyone who is stuck on a feeling.

Limeflower Always best used in a tea, limeflower takes the strain off the heart by helping you to relax and lower your blood pressure.

Cinnamon bark Renowned for bringing energy to the chest, cinnamon warms circulation and helps boost the heart. Its invigorating properties help keep the blood flowing and the emotions moving.

Motherwort Not just for mothers, motherwort is also known by herbalists as *Leonarus cardiaca*. Like a lion, motherwort is a heart tonic that brings you courage and confidence. Fluttering hearts become rhythmical and blood pressure can become normal.

Saffron Entering the heart channels, saffron lifts awareness and eases the strain of anger and depression. Traditionally used to help increase blood flow, its water-soluble carotenoids help to protect cell membranes, essential for a healthy heart.

Rose flower A specific for the heart. Its soft and gentle astringency strengthens tissues and holds them in place, helping to prevent weaknesses and pain. Rose's essential oils ease anger and bring joy.

Pomegranate juice This amazing sweet and sour juice is packed with artery-protecting antioxidants.

Bliss of the gods

Theobroma cacao is known to us as cocoa (or once there's some sugar and fat in there, chocolate). Theobroma means 'food of the gods' – and with good reason. Try this elixir for an entirely new and extremely decadent experience.

Unsweetened chocolate 100g/3½oz
Water or nut milk 100ml/3½fl oz
Vanilla bean essence 1–2 drops to taste
Honey to taste

This will serve 2 small cups of bliss-inducing nectar.

Melt the chocolate in a bain-marie before stirring in the water or nut milk. Add the vanilla bean essence and honey to taste then pour into small coffee cups. Words aren't fit to describe the next few seconds of your life…

Play around with this recipe. Add a drop of orange essential oil or some rose water to transform it into an entirely different experience.

Unsweetened chocolate Cacao is very rich in flavonoids that have strong antioxidant properties. These flavonoids have an astringent flavour, which is why sugar and fat are added to make chocolate smooth. They may be astringent, but flavonoids from cacao (similar to those found in red wine and tea) have been shown to significantly reduce risk of cardiovascular disease. And rather like caffeine in tea, the theobromine in cacao is mildly stimulating.

But the best thing about cacao is the neurotransmitter anandamide, known as the bliss chemical (*anand* is the Hindi word for 'bliss'). Cacao kisses our anandamide receptors and initiates feelings of bliss. Cannabis initiates the same feelings. So does orgasm. And just to prove that nature loves us being happy, cacao also contains enzyme inhibitors that slow the breakdown of anandamide. This means that the anandamide we naturally produce may remain longer within the brain when we consume cacao, prolonging blissful and euphoric feelings.

Cacao is also a useful source of the antispasmodic mineral magnesium. The pain-relieving and mood-balancing high magnesium content may explain why women crave chocolate during menstruation.

Vanilla bean essence Vanilla is an essential part of this elixir. The flavour molecules in vanilla open the vanilloid receptors on our tongue that help us experience taste and flavour, so adding vanilla to chocolate means we can enjoy chocolate more intensely and for longer. Other compounds in clove, cinnamon and ginger do this too. Of course, vanilla is an exotic expression of sweet bliss – when it combines with honey, it creates true harmony.

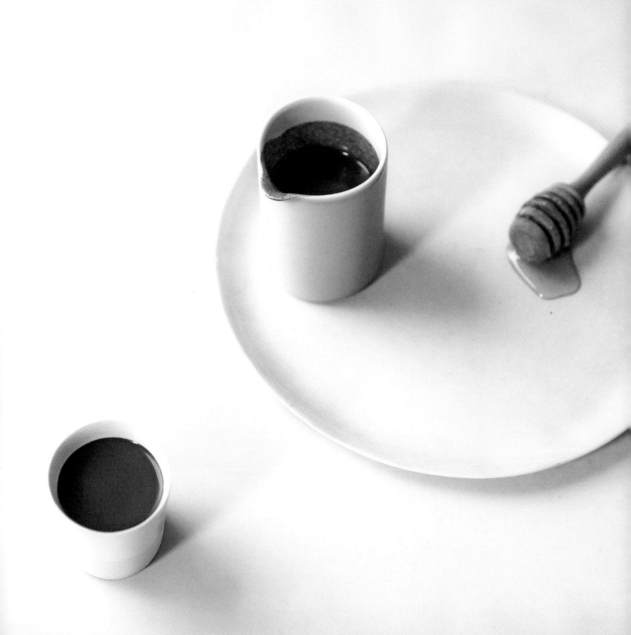

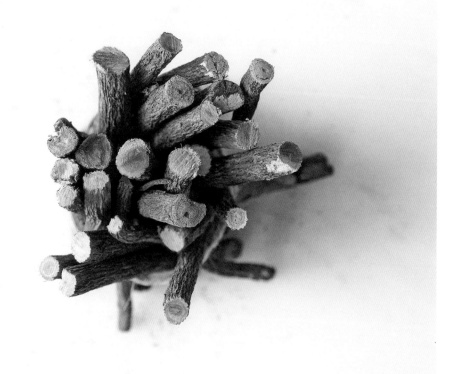

Sweetness in a cup. Favoured by Buddhist monks for attaining peace and clarity. I drink it every day.

Sweet licorice

Licorice root 5g

This will serve 2–3 cups of natural nectar.

Put the licorice root in a pot.
Add 500ml/18fl oz freshly boiled filtered water. Leave to steep for 5–10 minutes, then strain.

Licorice root Licorice root is one of my favourite plants. I prescribe it to most of my patients and include it in many of our Pukka teas. Licorice is traditionally used to bring a formula together by harmonising any extremes. It balances the big flavours and effects of other ingredients in the herbal teas. It works a bit like a pinch of salt in your food, drawing out and marrying the flavours. Because of this quality, licorice is considered to enhance the power of synergy between the different herbs in a blend leading to a more positive effect (see p19). I always think of licorice when there is weakness, dryness or heat in the body, specifically in the lungs, digestive system and nervous system – it can help a dry cough, acidic digestion or fatigue and burn-out. And it can increase overall vitality.

From an Ayurvedic point of view, licorice is sweet, soft, *demulcent*, protective and rejuvenating. It helps to calm the *vata* nervous system and clear excess *pitta* heat, but can increase *kapha* fluids. In modern herbalism it is used as an *adaptogen*, anti-inflammatory, anti-dyspeptic, anti-ulcer, *expectorant*, anti-hepatotoxic, antiviral and antibacterial. Its specific effect on the adrenal system points to its beneficial effect on cortisol.

You may have heard that licorice isn't safe for everyone all of the time – it is worth explaining this and clarifying any confusions.

Continued overleaf

Joy & Happiness

Sweet licorice

The safety of using any herb is influenced by who is taking it, how much they are taking, what form they are taking it in, and when they are taking it. In the context of this recipe, and when used sensibly, licorice is completely safe. Reports of issues with licorice largely relate to people eating large amounts of licorice sweets (over 500g per day over a period of some time) – these sweets also contain high levels of sugar and salt.

That aside, the main thing to understand about the safety of licorice is that it contains the triterpenoid saponin glycyrrhizic acid (GA). This is a natural plant molecule that gives licorice its sweet taste, as well as bringing many of its therapeutic benefits. There is a small chance that high levels of GA used over a long period of time can effect electrolyte balance in the body, so some caution is warranted. At very high levels it can cause retention of sodium, which can raise blood pressure. When used as a whole herb (as we do in Pukka teas) rather than an isolated extract, licorice has constituents that counter this effect. Nonetheless, it is best to avoid licorice if you have hypertension. And don't consume too much if you are pregnant. As a rule of thumb, 3g a day is fine for everyone and 1.5g a day if you are pregnant.

So, licorice is sweet, harmonising, rejuvenating, effective and sustainable (when harvested in the right way). It's also safe for everyone who uses it sensibly.

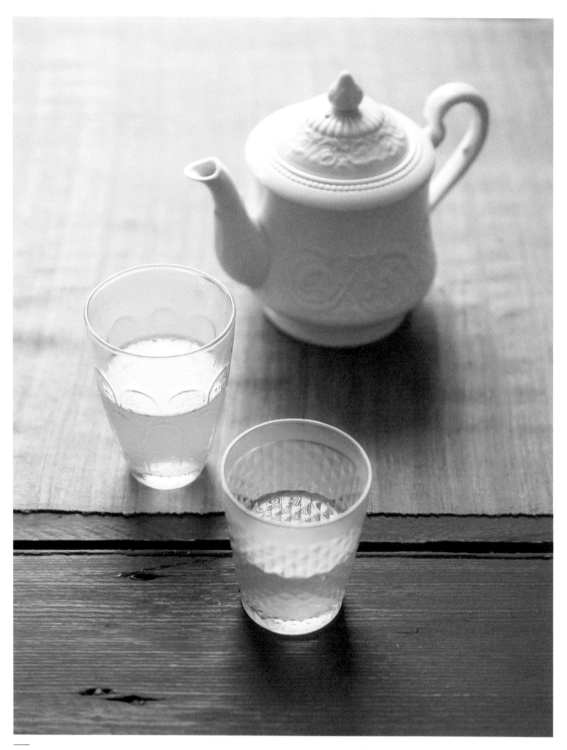

Light on tulsi

This is a wonderfully simple cup of tea that shines a bit of light into your life.

Tulsi leaf 5g

This will serve 2 cups of instant happiness.

Put the tulsi leaves in a pot. Add 500ml/ 18fl oz freshly boiled filtered water. Leave to steep for 5–10 minutes, then strain and let the light glow.

Tulsi leaf This leafy member of the mint family has an aromatic warmth. When used as a hot infusion it increases circulation, helps digestion and increases the digestive fire. It can be very useful to drink if you are feeling the start of a cold – it can blow it away. Its essential oils and ursolic acid content are associated with its ability to modulate inflammation, reduce infections and help regulate a healthy cell cycle. Its dispersing action makes it very useful for protecting from seasonal malaise as it reduces stagnant *kapha* and cold *vata*.

Hindus grow it outside their houses to 'cleanse' the outdoor space before someone enters their home. And in Ayurveda, this is a tea that lifts the life-force to the exterior and cleanses your 'inner space'. It's a favourite of yoga enthusiasts for its ability to raise the spirits and lift your mood. Tulsi really lets the light in.

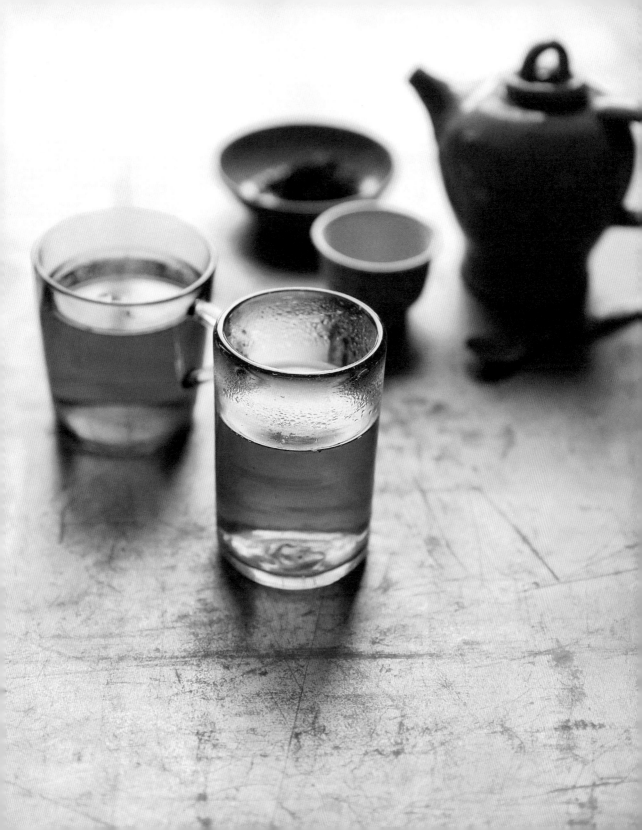

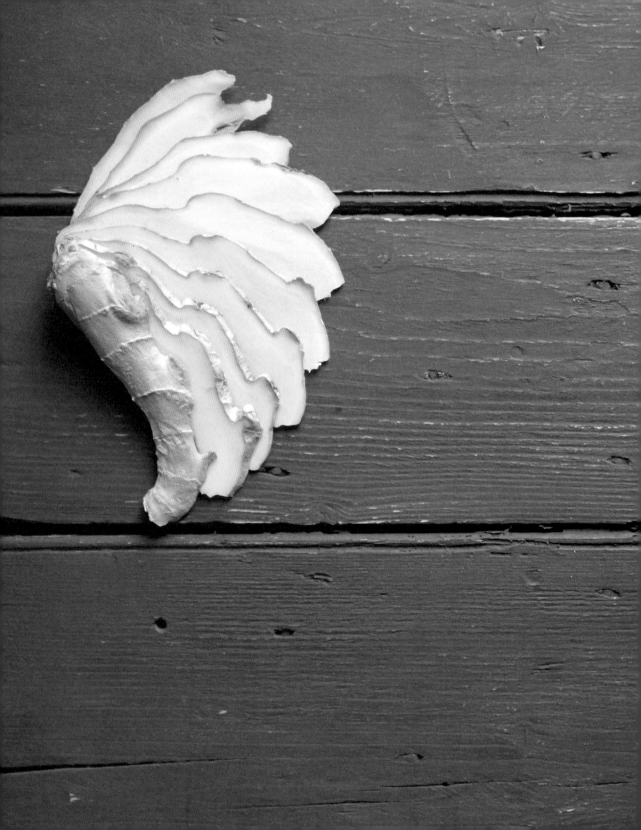

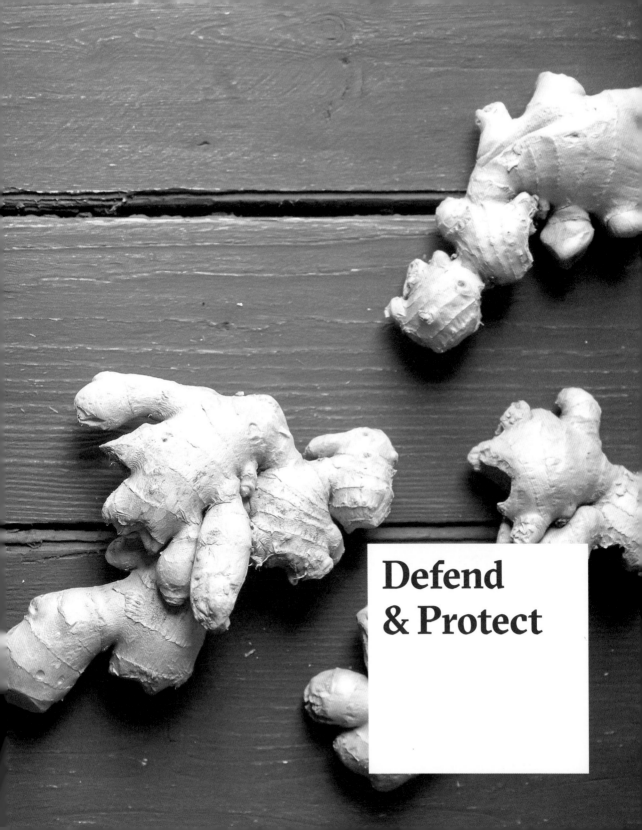

Defend
& Protect

"It is immunity (ojas) which keeps all living beings refreshed. There can be no life without strong immunity."
Ayurveda doctor Charaka, from Charaka Samhita written some 2,000 years ago

Here are some of my favourite teas for nipping a cold in the bud and supporting the immune system. Our immunity does a lot of work – it is essentially our natural protective response to infections and inflammations.

Luckily, nature is ready to help as plants are packed with antimicrobial and immune enhancing compounds. And the miracle is, unlike antibiotics, they haven't become less effective over time. Our use of thousands of plants over millennia suggests that bacteria, fungi and viruses have less ability to develop resistance to a broad-spectrum botanical pharmacy than to the narrow pharmaceutical one used in our modern health system.

The herbs used in these teas are some of the species that have been relied upon for generations for their protective and curative effects. They will help everyone in the family keep seasonal lurgies, sore throats, chesty coughs and aches and pains at bay.

On a deeper level, the immune system maintains the relationship between our mind-body-spirit and the world in which we live. Our immunity is wonderfully multi-dimensional and requires nourishment from diverse sources including digestive, emotional, psychological and hormonal. One way of looking at how our immunity functions is to think about how well we can digest our life. Ayurveda talks about how we can assimilate the challenges that life throws at us, be it an indulgent birthday feast, some bad news or a nasty bug that's going around. The herbs in this chapter are here to help.

For gram to teaspoon conversion see p24

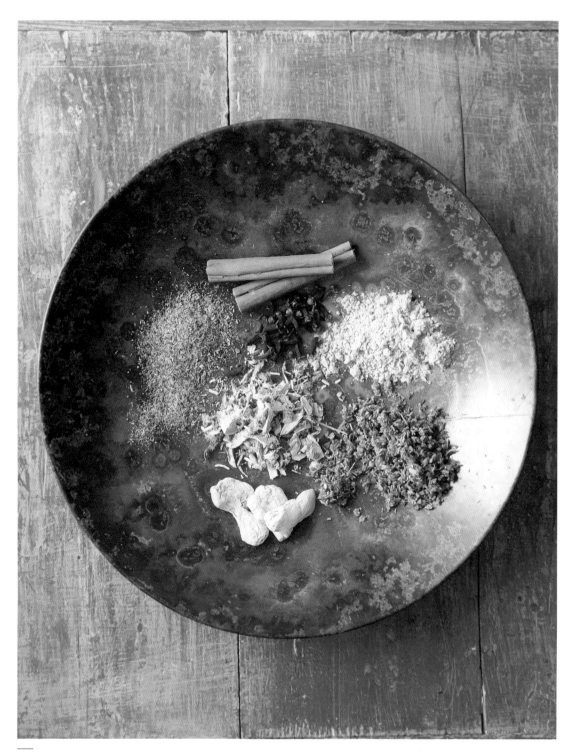

Sing a song

This is a sweet and silky tea to soothe a sore throat, rid you of the croak and let you sing a song. Use it when you have been singing, talking or living it up a bit too much.

Marshmallow root 3g
Marshmallow leaf 3g
Licorice root 2g
Ginger root powder 2g
Cinnamon bark 2g
Cloves 2g
Slippery elm bark powder 1g per cup (please note this is a threatened species so only buy from a verified sustainable and organic source)
Manuka honey a dash per cup

This will serve 2–3 cups of melody-making tea.

Put the marshmallow root and leaf in a cup with 200ml cold water and leave overnight (the root's mucilage is best extracted in cold water). The next day, put the remaining ingredients (except for the slippery elm bark and honey) in a pot. Add 400ml freshly boiled filtered water. Leave to steep for 10–15 minutes, then strain both liquids and combine to make the final herbal tea. Add the slippery elm bark powder and a dash of honey to each cup before stirring in the tea.

Marshmallow root and leaf Soft, sweet and a true hug-in-a-cup herb, marshmallow oozes soothing mucilage that helps clear a raspy voice. Any stuck phlegm will be loosened by marshmallow's softening power.

Licorice root This is a singer's favourite as it nourishes the vocal cords and strengthens the lungs. It literally sweetens your voice.

Ginger root Easing the flow of your breathing, ginger's warming qualities help bring force and gusto back into your voice.

Cinnamon bark Strong and bold, cinnamon bark is excellent at encouraging circulation in your chest. A sip of cinnamon is like taking in a deep breath.

Cloves Having a direct affinity with the throat, potent clove essential oils help your voice soar to new heights.

Slippery elm bark Nature's throat-loving herb lubricates dryness and softens a croak to a purr.

Manuka honey This is a good friend to the lungs. Honey directs all the other herbs to the source of the voice, helping to strengthen with softness. Manuka makes the honey that bit more antibacterial to help resist any lurking lurgies.

Defend & Protect

Breathe

A fresh and uplifting tea to awaken your lungs and help you breathe. Use this if you have a cough, are feeling tight-chested, or you just want to relish the joy of breathing a bit more deeply.

Lemongrass leaf 4g
Thyme leaf 3g
Tulsi leaf 3g
Ginger root powder 2g
Aniseed 2g
Peppermint oil 1 drop
Honey to taste

This will serve 2–3 cups of lung-nourishing tea.

Put all of the ingredients (except for the honey) in a pot. Add 500ml/18fl oz freshly boiled filtered water. Leave to steep for 10–15 minutes, then strain. Add a dash of honey to taste.

You can use this tea as a steam inhalation as well. Put the herbs in a large bowl, add boiled water, put a towel over your head and around the bowl so no steam leaks out. Breathe this in for 5 minutes and your respiration will be radically transformed.

Lemongrass leaf Beautifully aromatic, this fragrant grass showers the senses and encourages them to wake up. Its citrus zing opens your lungs and helps you to breathe.

Thyme leaf Thyme is magic for the lungs: it brings strength and helps open where there is mucus and obstruction.

Tulsi leaf In Ayurveda, this sacred leaf is full of *prana*, which helps to bring the breath of life. It has a natural ability to move your energy upwards and outwards, helping to dilate the bronchioles and let the air in and out. If you don't have tulsi, replace it with basil.

Ginger root Stimulating ginger lends a warming heat that opens up your chest. The pungent essential oils are also good at clearing phlegm.

Aniseed A specific tonic for the lungs, aniseed helps to remove stuck mucus. A low digestive fire is often the cause of this lung congestion, so by kindling your digestive fire, warming aniseed helps to remove the tendency of getting bunged-up, treating the root of the problem.

Peppermint oil Peppermint leaf has about 1 per cent essential oil, so when it's made into a pure oil it is extremely concentrated and far more intense than the fresh leaves. It opens and clears the head and nasal passages.

Honey Honey helps carry the other herbs to where they need to act in the lungs.

Defend & Protect

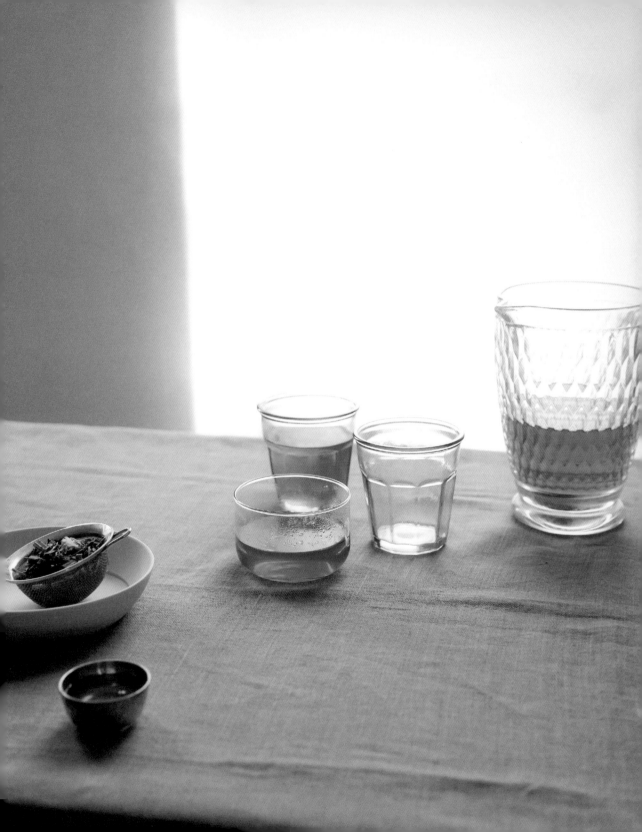

This tempting, fruity berry blend is revitalising and warming – the perfect support come winter storms. It targets the cause of seasonal infections by strengthening both short- and long-term immunity.

Elderberry & echinacea winter warmer

Echinacea root 2g
Elderberry 2g
Elderflower 2g
Rosehip 2g
Peppermint leaf 2g
Orange peel 2g
Aniseed 1g
Ginger root powder 1g
Licorice root 1g
Orange essential oil a drop per cup

This will serve 2 cups of good health.

Put all of the ingredients (except for the orange essential oil) in a pot. Add 500ml/18fl oz freshly boiled filtered water. Leave to steep for 10–15 minutes, then strain. Add a drop of orange essential oil to each cup.

Echinacea root Aromatic, tongue-tingling, bittersweet echinacea root boosts your body's immune system. A renowned blood cleanser, it's traditionally used to heal blood-poisoning from snake bites. It contains stimulating and warming properties that enhance general vitality.

Elderberry Sweet, plump, purple-black elderberry is a delicious way to boost your immune system. Its cell protectors are famed for their lung-strengthening antiviral properties. Elderberry's colourful purple pigments are packed with antioxidants.

Elderflower Helps to cleanse toxins by encouraging your body's natural response, which is to induce mild sweating and clear mucus. Its creamy clusters of unusually fragranced flowers can be used for pure healing (to ease colds and fevers) or for pure pleasure (to make wine, champagne and cordial).

Rosehip Ripe, red and refreshing, rosehip offers gentle support for your immune system. Famed for supplementing Vitamin C, this nourishing hip also delivers bioflavonoids and other protective nutrients.

Peppermint leaf Its uplifting menthol vapours clear your head and removes congestion – it also supports the elderflower's mild sweat-inducing effects. In Ayurveda, it opens up your channels so your life-force's healing vitality can move where it needs to.

Continued overleaf

Defend & Protect

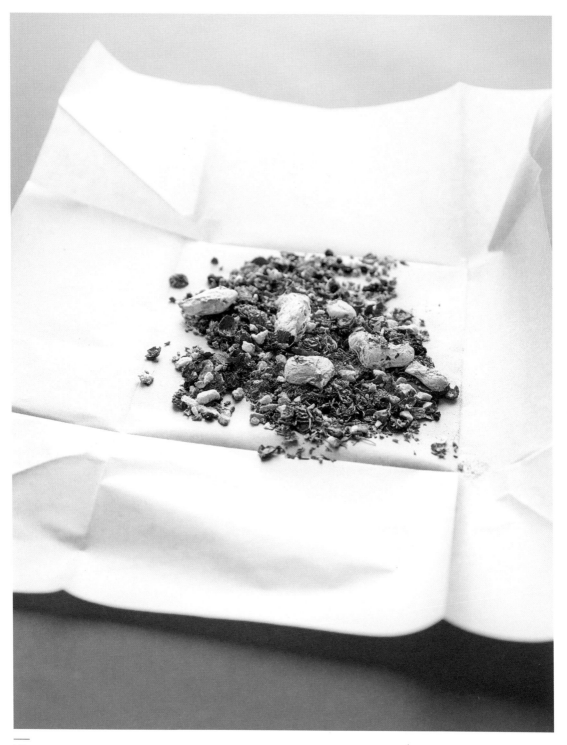

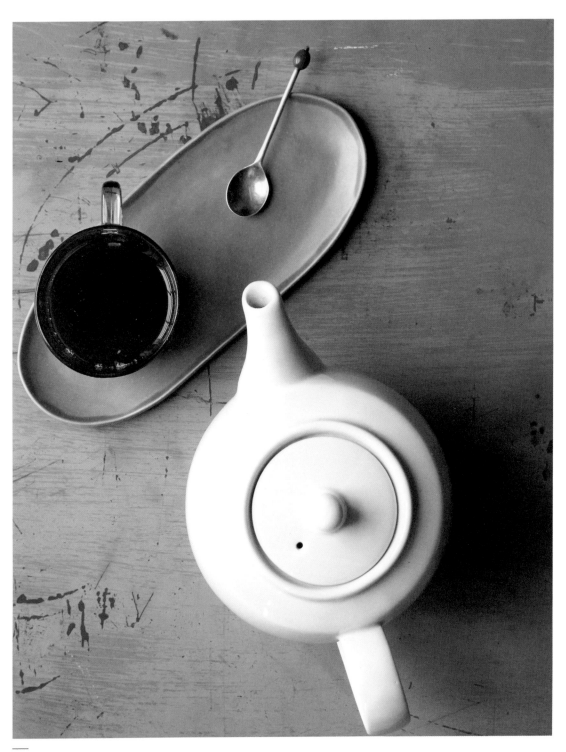

Elderberry & echinacea winter warmer

Orange peel Brimming with colourful pigments and lovely essential oils, orange peel has a time-tested reputation for cutting through the stifling effects of winter damp from a bunged-up nose to phlegmy chest.

Aniseed Working with orange peel, aniseed is held in high regard by herbalists for its *expectorant* action, which clears the chest of excess mucus.

Ginger root Warming metabolism and improving overall circulation, ginger takes your vitality up a couple of notches.

Licorice root Moistening licorice provides a soothing balm for dry, irritated tissues, helping to clear stuck mucus from the lungs.

Orange essential oil Fragrant sweet orange warms and revives, and helps lift dampened spirits.

Elderberry elixir

This syrup is also known as Elderberry Rob and should be an essential store-cupboard elixir in every house. It's easy to make, enjoyable to drink and a great keep-me-healthy-through-winter herbal remedy.

Fresh elderberry 1kg/35oz
Clove bud 10 buds
Cinnamon bark 3 quills
Fresh ginger root 10g, about
    5cm/2in piece
Sugar 250g/9oz

Collect your fresh berries on an autumn day. Wash and destalk the berries by using a fork as a mini rake. It's a rather satisfying job as the berries pop off their stalks. Put the elderberries in a pan with 1 cup of water and simmer until the berries have released most of their juices. Place a sieve over a bowl, pour the berries and the liquid into the sieve and crush the berries with a fork to help strain as much liquid as possible into the bowl. Pour this juice back in the saucepan. Add the remaining ingredients. Simmer for 30 minutes on a low heat. Strain again over a bowl. And then decant into sterilised bottles and tightly seal. Store in the fridge for up to 6 months. To drink, add 2 tbsp of Elderberry elixir to a cup of hot water.

Elderberry Elderberries have a time-honoured reputation as one of the great lung tonics, which is especially valued in the damp cold of northern Europe and the Americas. These dark-purple berries are a rich source of Vitamin C, anthocyanins and flavonoids, all of which are powerful antioxidants that protect the body from immune-damaging free radicals. Elderberries have a strong affinity with the respiratory system and encourage the process of expectoration, reducing acute and chronic mucus congestion. Their sweet juices are incredibly soothing and coat the mucous membranes, alleviating sore throats and irritating coughs. Elderberries have also been shown to halt a virus's ability to proliferate (by neutralising the neuraminidase enzyme, which many flu drugs target) and prevent viral replication in the respiratory mucous membranes. Amazingly, it neutralises ten strains of flu virus. Use elderberry at the first sign of contact.
The spices Cloves, cinnamon and ginger all add warming and stimulating effects that help to reinvigorate your energy. They help you ward off the cold from the inside out, bringing you a wonderful winter-warming glow.

If you don't want to add sugar then skip that step. Instead, pour the sugar-free juice into some ice-cube trays and store in the freezer. When you want a cup just pop the juice-cube out, add hot water and a little honey to sweeten.

Defend & Protect

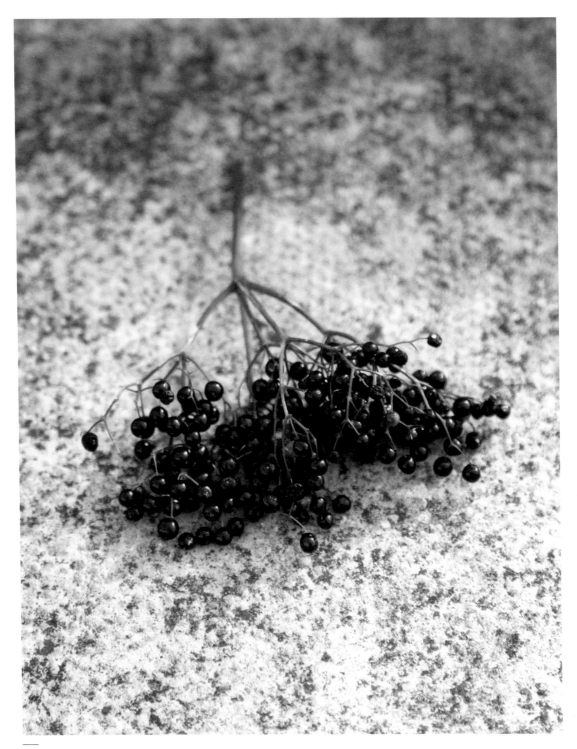

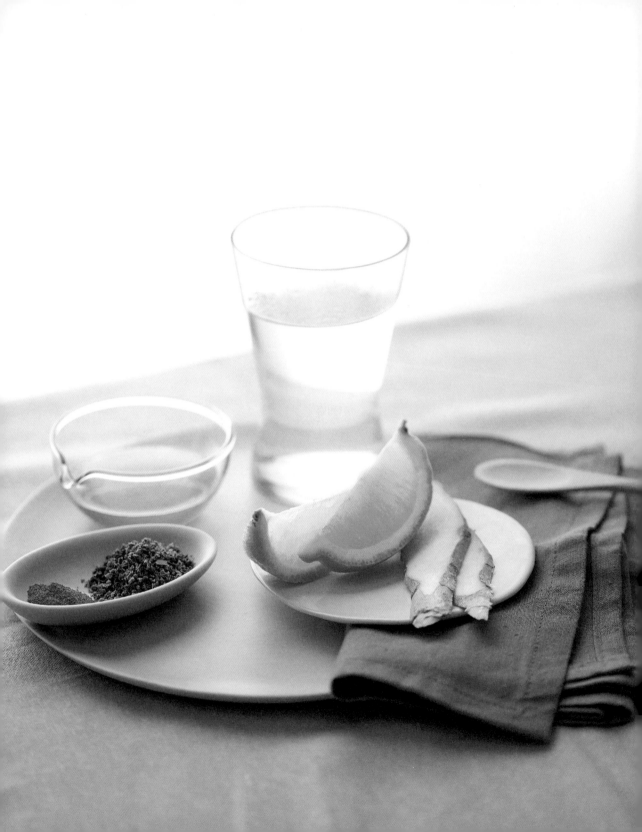

This is one of the great herbal tea classics, and thanks to my mum, one of the first ones I ever sipped. I have slightly tweaked the recipe so it's more beneficial for fighting lurgies. Use it if you have a chill or feel a bit under the weather.

Lemon & ginger with manuka honey

Fresh ginger root 10g, about 5cm/2in
Elderflower 4g
Turmeric root powder 1g
Lemon juice a twist per cup
Manuka honey 1 tsp per cup

This will serve 2 cups of a herbal classic.

Grate the ginger and put it in a pot with the rest of the ingredients except the lemon and honey. Add 500ml/18fl oz freshly boiled filtered water. Leave to steep for 5–10 minutes, then strain. Add the lemon and honey to each cup.

Ginger root The wonderful, digestion-aiding ginger boosts circulation and takes the body's vitality up a couple of notches. Its stimulating warmth lends a subtle spicy tang.
Elderflower Light and purifying, these summer blossoms help to cleanse by increasing circulation to the periphery, which induces a very mild sweat, helping to halt the spread of any seasonal viruses.
Turmeric root A close relative of ginger, the golden super-spice turmeric is relied on in India as a gentle herbal antibiotic useful for infections. It also makes this tea look like liquid gold.
Lemon juice Pleasingly mouth-watering, lemon juice adds a refreshing tang to the tea and cuts through stuck mucus. Lemons are packed with natural Vitamin C and immune-enhancing bioflavonoids that both taste and do good.
Manuka honey Sweet, soothing and nourishing, manuka honey combines the therapeutic benefits of honey with the antimicrobial qualities of the manuka tree. This is a natural powerhouse in a pot.

At the first sign of a cold, look to this classic formula. Bacteria and viruses are most active at lower body temperatures, so we get fevers or 'temperatures' in response to our immune system's effort to reduce microbial overload. This blend helps your immune system fight back.

Incredible immunity

Yarrow top 3g
Peppermint leaf 3g
Elderflower 3g
Tulsi leaf 3g
Fresh ginger root 3g, about 1½cm/⅝in

This will serve 2–3 cups of flu-free freedom.

Put all of the ingredients in a pot. Add 500ml/18fl oz freshly boiled filtered water. Leave to steep for 5–10 minutes, then strain. Drink while it's piping hot.

Yarrow top An incredible herb that invigorates circulation right to the tips of your toes. Yarrow is used to release the muscular tension that comes hand-in-hand with an infection. Its botanical name is *Achillea millefolium*, as it's also great for healing your Achilles heel, which in this case is a challenged immune system. It tastes very herbal.

Peppermint leaf When used in a hot cup of tea, the essential oils in peppermint help diffuse tension in the periphery, encouraging a mild sweat. It is a gentle, stimulating *diaphoretic*.

Elderflower One of the great relaxing *diaphoretic* herbs, elderflowers help open up the pores in the surface of the skin by reducing resistance in the capillaries so that blood can move to the surface and help you cool down.

Tulsi leaf Tulsi is India's favourite panacea for fevers. It is warming, relaxing, ascendant, helps to raise spirits, increase body temperature and encourages a mild sweat to throw the flu out.

Ginger root A warming and stimulating *diaphoretic*, essential in all teas blended for stimulating a sweat. Dry ginger works too, but fresh ginger is more specific for spreading out to the peripheral edges.

Defend & Protect

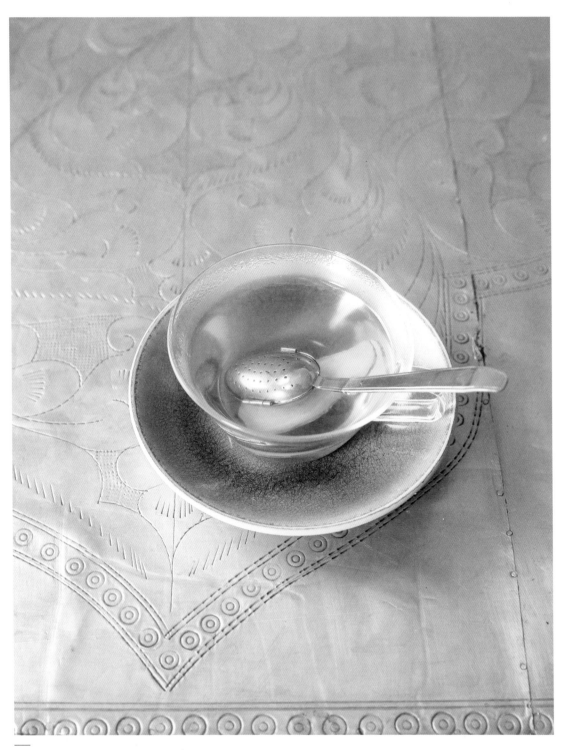

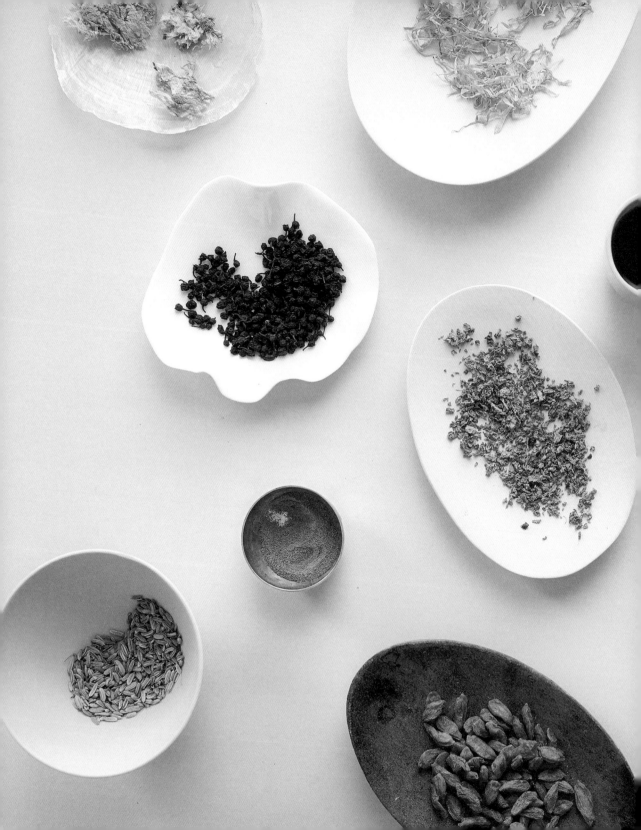

These herbs are potent eye-lovers. They all feed the brilliance of the eyes, helping to protect and enhance your vision. As well as reducing tired and dry eyes, this tea will help them sparkle.

Eagle eyes

Goji berry 3g
Chrysanthemum flower 2g
Bilberry 2g
Amla powder 2g
Marigold (calendula) petal 2g
Fennel seed 2g
Turmeric root powder 1g
Blueberry concentrate 1 tsp per
    cup (or blackcurrant
    concentrate or
    Elderberry Elixir p144)

This will serve 2–3 cups of eye-nourishing elixir.

Put all of the ingredients (except for the blueberry concentrate) in a pot. Add 500ml/18fl oz freshly boiled filtered water. Leave to steep for 5–10 minutes, then strain. Add 1 tsp blueberry concentrate to each cup.

If you can't find blueberry concentrate then use blackcurrant concentrate instead. In fact, anything potently purple will do.

Goji berry Known as *gou qi zi* in China, this little red berry is packed with beta-carotene that converts into Vitamin A, helping to feed the eye. It has long been used for failing eyesight and dry eyes.

Chrysanthemum flower This little flower even looks like an eye! It helps to bring brightness and clarity to your vision. Good for bloodshot eyes.

Bilberry Brimming with eye-protecting anthocyanins, bilberries are lauded for promoting penetrating sight and good night vision. Valued for their ability to protect capillary integrity, bilberries help circulation in the eye.

Amla One of Ayurveda's most respected optical herbs, amla cleanses, protects and rejuvenates, which is just what every eye needs.

Marigold petal High in lutein and zeaxanthin, two important carotenoids for eye health, marigold petal helps to feed the macula ensuring laser-like vision.

Fennel seed This sweet little beauty is used to help you see with clarity – the potent antioxidant power of its essential oils help to protect eyesight from decline.

Turmeric root A powerful circulation invigorator, turmeric helps to take blood to the eyes, bringing important nutrition to the seat of vision. Turmeric works synergistically with the other herbs in this blend to supercharge their powerful antioxidant activity. A lack of antioxidants in the diet is associated with cataracts and macular degeneration, two vision problems we want to avoid.

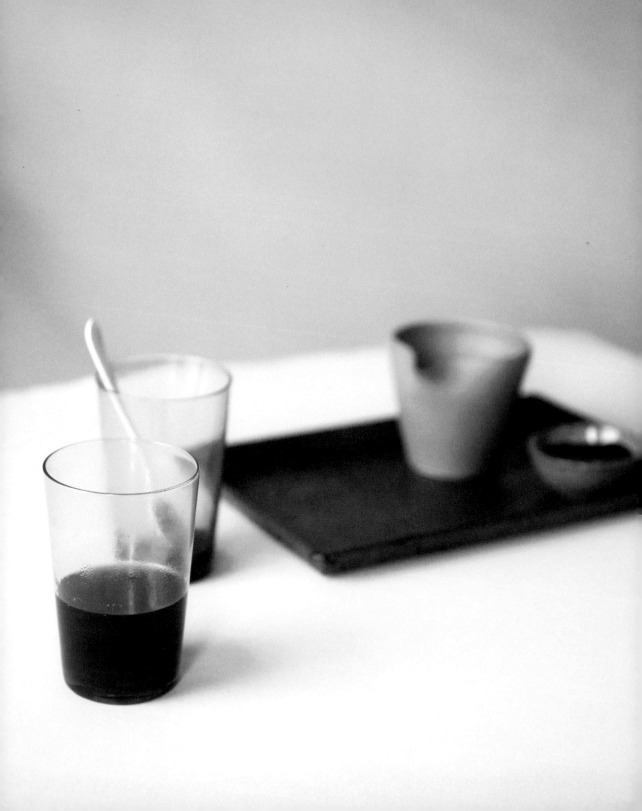

Thick, long, lustrous and flowing hair is the epitome of youthful good health. Use these herbs to help your hair stay strong, maintain its natural colour and keep it blowing in the wind.

Illustriously lustrous locks

Horsetail 6g
Nettle leaf 10g/⅓oz
Bhringraj leaf 4g
Rosemary 2g
Molasses 1 tsp per cup

This will serve 2–3 cups of a lock-loving tea.

Put the horsetail in a saucepan with 200ml/7fl oz cold filtered water. Bring to the boil and allow to simmer for 30 minutes to make sure you extract as many of the minerals as possible. Add the remaining ingredients (except for the molasses) and 400ml/14fl oz freshly boiled filtered water to the pan. Leave to steep for 30 minutes, strain and add 1 tsp molasses to each cup.

Horsetail This plant even looks like hair. It's high in minerals, which are best extracted by boiling the silica-rich herb in water first.
Nettle leaf Nettle is food for your hair, but you need to consume a good amount for maximum mineral nourishment. Long used to delay greying hair and bring lustre and shine.
Bhringraj leaf A popular Ayurvedic herb meaning 'king of hair', this is used to help keep your tresses their natural colour and stop greying. It might be a little tricky to source this herb so just add more nettle if you need to replace it.
Rosemary Long regarded as having an affinity with the head, rosemary carries the nutritive benefits of the whole blend to the roots of the hairs.
Molasses This rich by-product from sugarcane is low in sucrose (as most of it has been syphoned off for sugar production) and high in Vitamin B6 and minerals such as iron, calcium and magnesium. It builds the blood and brings strength to your hair.

Use this tea as a hair rinse to treat dandruff, itchy scalp, greying and thinning hair. Make 1 cup to drink and 1 cup to rinse. After a shower, pour it on your hair and leave for a couple of hours before rinsing off.

Defend & Protect

Joint protector

It's almost an inevitable human condition that we will suffer from some sort of joint pain as we get older. All that wear-and-tear can catch up with us. These herbs will help keep the red-hot inflammation of arthritis and gout at bay.

Turmeric root powder 3g
Boswellia resin 2g
Ginger root powder 2g
Celery seed 2g
Ashwagandha root 1g
Licorice root 1g
Meadowsweet leaf 1g
Honey to taste

This will serve 2–3 cups of ache-free tea.

Put all of the ingredients (except for the meadowsweet leaf and honey) in a saucepan with 600ml/21fl oz cold filtered water. Cover with a lid and simmer for 15 minutes. Take off the heat and add the meadowsweet leaf. Leave to steep for 10 minutes, strain and add some honey to taste. I won't say enjoy, as it's a pretty heady brew, but you will appreciate the effects.

This also works as a foot soak or compress. Make the tea and then soak a flannel in the warm liquid, squeeze out the excess fluid and place over the affected part for 30 minutes. It brings swift and welcome relief. Do note that as the tea has turmeric in it, it will stain the flannel and anything it drips on.

Turmeric root This cuts the cause of joint pain off at its root by inhibiting the inflammatory pathways that make the joints swell and hurt. It's a safe alternative to NSAID paracetamol and aspirin. Long used in Ayurvedic and Chinese herbalism to invigorate blood and remove stagnation, turmeric works on multiple pathways (such as your hormones and immune system) at the same time to bring about remarkable results.

Boswellia resin A relative of frankincense, boswellia resin 'breaks' blockages (stiff joints) and eases the stiffness that so often causes pain. It 'scrapes' away the sticky-swellings (toxins) that can appear in arthritic conditions. It has also been shown to be of benefit to those suffering from osteoarthritis. It tastes a bit funky, so reduce the dose if you don't like it.

Ginger root God's gift to us all, ginger is renowned for thinning the blood, helping to hasten circulation and ease pain. Its warming, stimulating and detoxifying properties make it a valuable anti-inflammatory.

Celery seed A classic diuretic that carries inflammatory uric acid out of the body so it doesn't accumulate in the difficult-to-navigate junctions of the joints.

Ashwagandha root Full of strength and vigour, ashwagandha root is said to make you as strong as a stallion. It brings strength to your bones and joints as well as being an effective anti-inflammatory that supports healthy immunity.

Licorice root Sweet and nourishing, licorice root helps to balance the extreme notes of the other herbs, making them more palatable and more effective.

Meadowsweet leaf This common hedgerow beauty is also known as Queen of the Meadow. It contains salicylates that convert in the body to help balance pain. Its astringent tannins also protect the stomach from ulcers, as well as the damaging effects of aspirin.

Defend & Protect

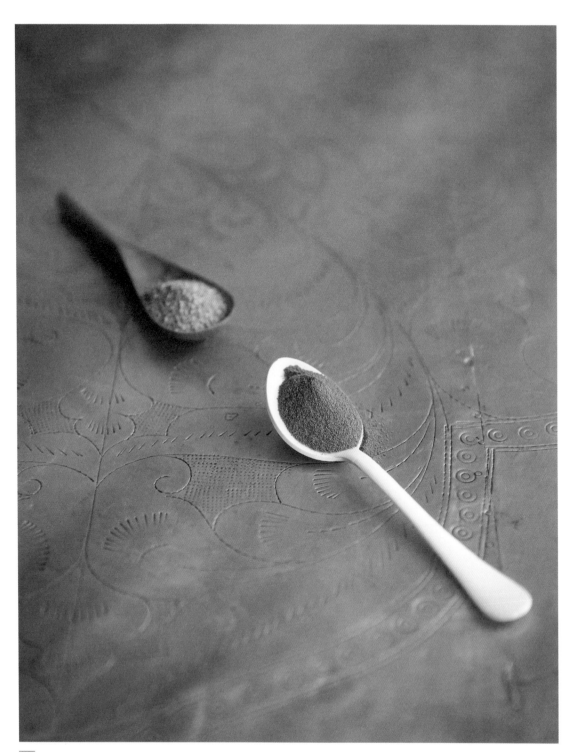

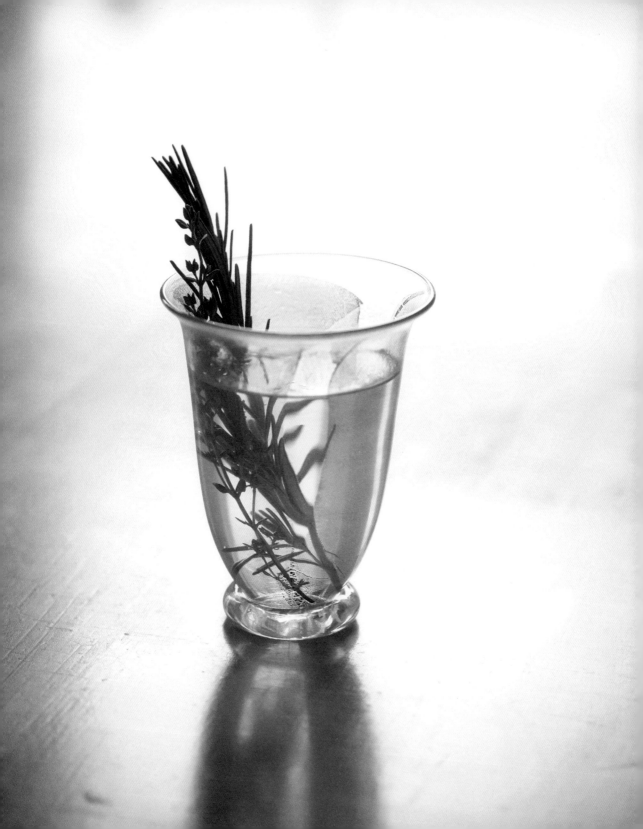

A gardener's classic, fit for a king. This is an easy tea to make with either bought fresh herbs or a few sprigs freshly picked from your garden. Life would not be the same without fresh rosemary and thyme. It's a great tea to make if you're feeling a bit stuffy in your chest or your head.

Rosemary & thyme

Fresh rosemary 1 sprig
Fresh thyme 1 sprig

Put the herbs in a cup. Add 250ml/9fl oz freshly boiled filtered water. Leave to steep for a few minutes, and enjoy with the herbs still in the cup.

Rosemary Research studies have shown that the essential oil from rosemary alleviates anxiety as well as improves cognition. As you drink it, you can feel it go to your head and wake you up. It also helps your digestive system and your liver's detoxification function – so, in a way, it removes burdens from your life. Rosemary is a spiritual herb in the sense that it helps raise your consciousness. It lightens the heavy feeling associated with the onset of a cold or a bout of low mood and tiredness.
Thyme Thyme is a warming, aromatic herb with a specific affinity with your chest. It helps you breathe deeply and puff your chest out so you are ready for what lies ahead. It has a potent antibacterial action that clears up chesty coughs. It clears phlegm so you can breathe more easily, as well as think more clearly.

Defend & Protect

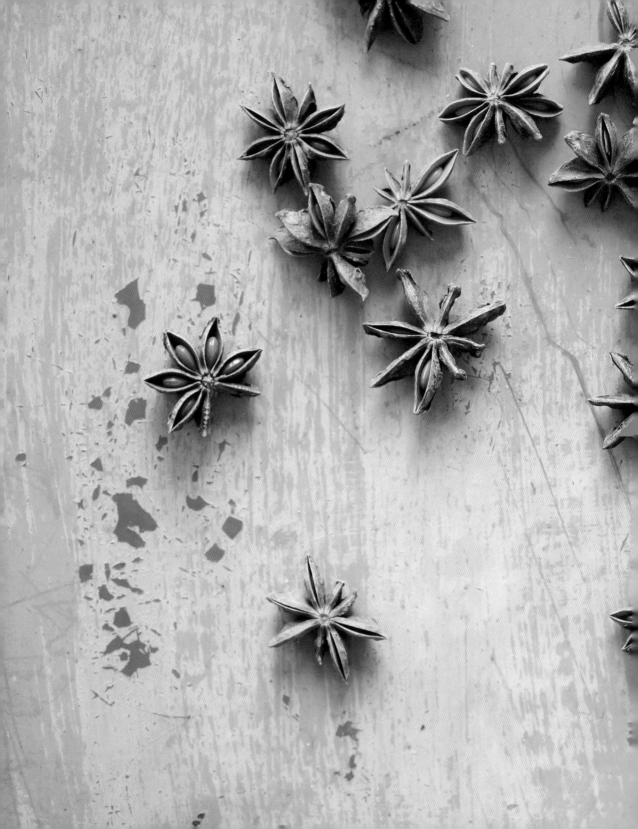

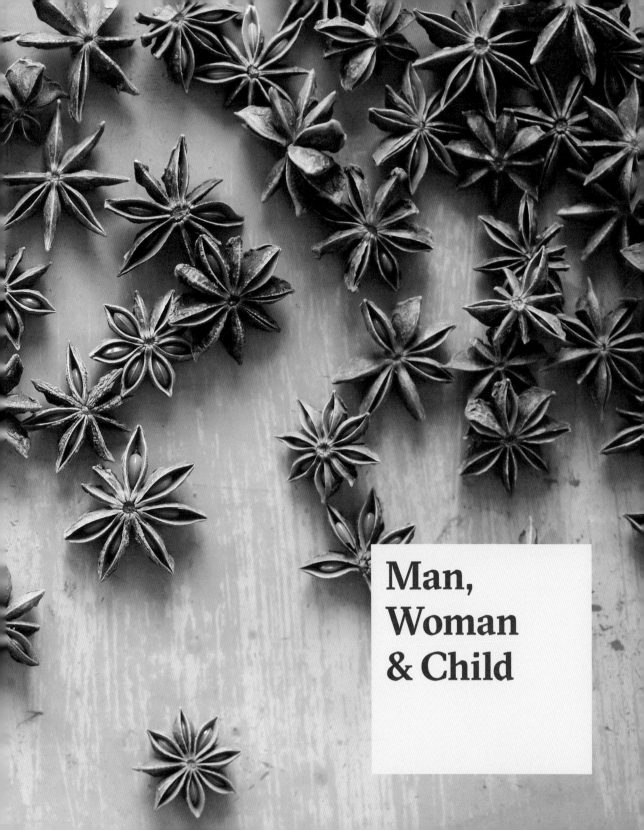

Man,
Woman
& Child

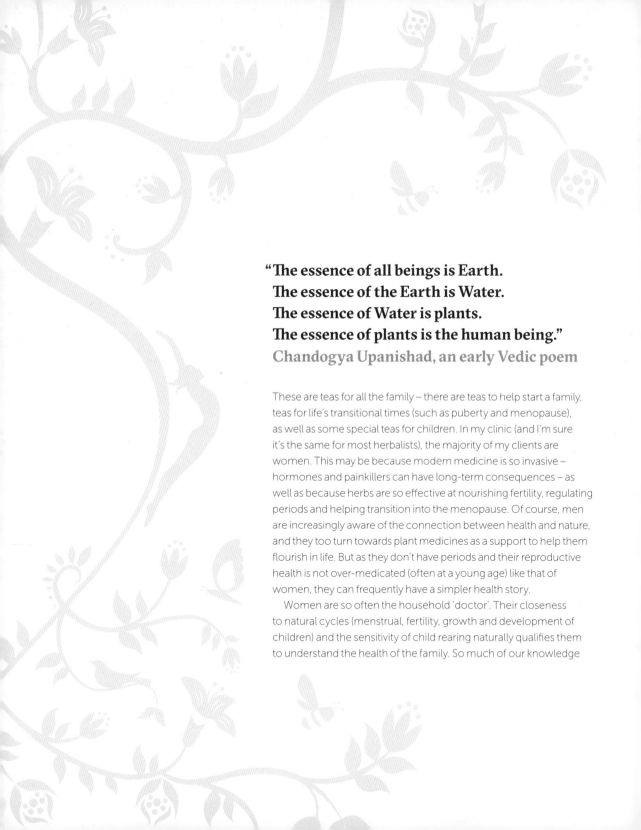

"The essence of all beings is Earth.
The essence of the Earth is Water.
The essence of Water is plants.
The essence of plants is the human being."
Chandogya Upanishad, an early Vedic poem

These are teas for all the family – there are teas to help start a family, teas for life's transitional times (such as puberty and menopause), as well as some special teas for children. In my clinic (and I'm sure it's the same for most herbalists), the majority of my clients are women. This may be because modern medicine is so invasive – hormones and painkillers can have long-term consequences – as well as because herbs are so effective at nourishing fertility, regulating periods and helping transition into the menopause. Of course, men are increasingly aware of the connection between health and nature, and they too turn towards plant medicines as a support to help them flourish in life. But as they don't have periods and their reproductive health is not over-medicated (often at a young age) like that of women, they can frequently have a simpler health story.

Women are so often the household 'doctor'. Their closeness to natural cycles (menstrual, fertility, growth and development of children) and the sensitivity of child rearing naturally qualifies them to understand the health of the family. So much of our knowledge of how plants heal is because women have carried this wisdom. Much of this traditional wisdom has been lost, but women (and men) have the opportunity to re-learn this crucial information.

Tea for children

If it wasn't so painful to see children suffer, treating their ailments would be a joy. Luckily, children's inherent sensitivity means they can quickly and positively respond to the gentle healing power of herbs. The more children get used to the taste and idea of herbs, the wider their palate and appreciation of nature becomes. It makes meal-times (and vegetable-eating) easier forever, and in this era of 'nature deficiency syndrome', that can only be a good thing. It is one of my favourite pleasures to see children select herbs and make tea. It's messy, amusing and full of surprises. As they get used to some of the more earthy flavours at an early age it helps them become more confident in exploring the marvels of nature as they grow up. At a young age they are open to connecting with the language of herbs and can then benefit from healing plants for the rest of their lives.

The children's teas are designed with 8–12 year-olds in mind. Divide the measure in half for 4–8 year-olds; and divide in quarter for 2–4 year-olds. Under 2s can have a few teaspoons. Seek the advice of a herbalist or doctor for any serious, concerning or lingering symptoms. See p25 for more on dosages for children of different ages and body weights.

For gram to teaspoon conversion see p24

This tea reaches deep into the reproductive system, nourishing our procreative and sexual energy. Use it when preparing for a family or for nurturing your love life. For men and women, this elixir feeds sex hormone release, improves egg/sperm quality and enhances orgasmic experiences.

Aphrodite's aphrodisiac

Shatavari root 4g
Ashwagandha root 2g
Licorice root 2g
Cinnamon bark 2g
Milk (any type) 250ml/9fl oz
Damiana leaf 2g
Cacao powder 1 tsp per cup
Maca root 1 tsp per cup
Flower pollen ½ tsp per cup
Vanilla essence a dash per cup
Honey (or Amaretto) a drop per cup

Makes 2 cups of the most amorous elixir.

Put the shatavari, ashwagandha, licorice and cinnamon in a saucepan with the milk and 250ml/9fl oz cold filtered water. Cover, bring to the boil and allow to simmer for 15 minutes. Take off the heat and add the damiana leaf. Leave to steep for 10 minutes, then strain. To each cup, add the cacao, maca, flower pollen, vanilla essence and honey. Then top with the tea and stir.

These herbs are rejuvenating tonics: they are sweet in taste, build your strength and replenish your sexual appetite. They specifically nourish fertility, enhance libido and strengthen your sexual organs.

Shatavari root In India, shatavari colloquially means 'she who has 100 husbands', referring to its ability to help a woman have an active sexual and reproductive life. It's traditionally used to increase breast size, enhance lubrication and optimise libido. Use it whenever there is a lack in desire, delayed orgasm or dryness. Or just for fun. As herbs are not sexist, it's also an effective male tonic where it performs similar strengthening stunts, increasing sperm count and quality.

Ashwagandha root Said to bring you the 'essence of a stallion', ashwagandha has legendary powers, enhancing stamina, erectile strength and libido. It brings grace, beauty and emotional sensitivity to both men and women. However, it's no herbal Viagra. Sexual nourishment cannot be replenished with a one-pill wonder. It's something that needs to be addressed in all aspects of your life: ashwagandha is only one part of that plan.

Damiana leaf This South American herb is used when loss of libido leads to feeling low. As a valuable restorative to the nervous system, it helps you relax into the moment.

Maca root Growing high in the Andes, maca root improves mental acuity, physical endurance, vitality and stamina. It's also a well known Peruvian aphrodisiac tonic for both men and women: it is used to increase libido as well improve sperm and egg health.

Flower pollen Flower pollen is a renowned energy nutrient, high in essential proteins and amino acids. Gathered by bees from fertile flowers, pollen is the source of life itself and represents all of nature's procreative potential.

Cinnamon, licorice, cacao and vanilla These aphrodisiacs invigorate circulation, strengthen your adrenals and evoke your erotic side. Honey and amaretto add a special touch of the taste of love: sweetness.

Man, Woman & Child

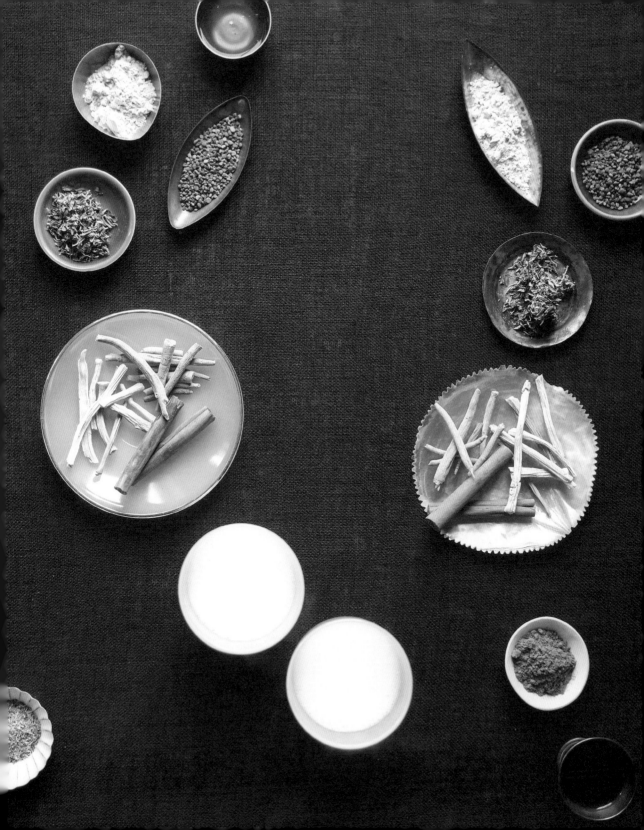

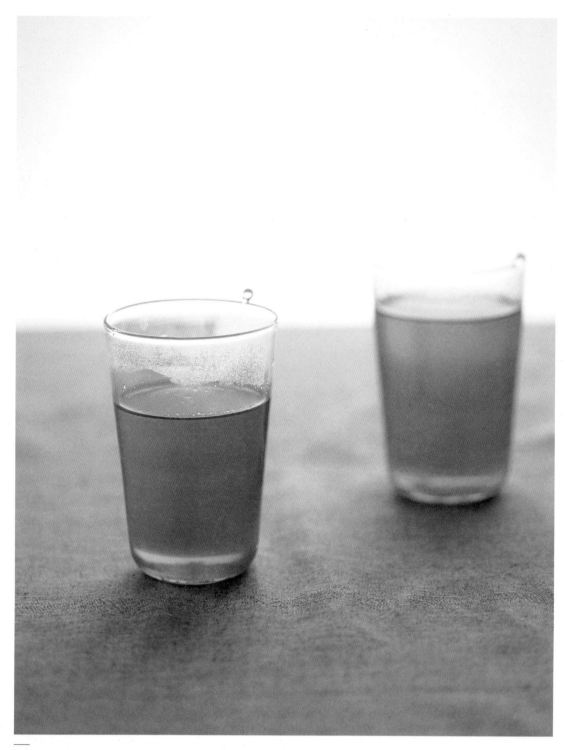

Moon balance

Everything will change, that at least is guaranteed. This tea is here to help you ease through the fluctuations within your monthly reproductive cycle. Drink it every day for a smooth lunar circumambulation.

Chamomile flower 3g
Shatavari root 2g
Hibiscus flower 2g
Dandelion root 2g
Rose flower 1g
Licorice root 1g
Vanilla pod 2cm/¾in cut up

This will serve 2–3 cups of perfect balance.

Put all of the ingredients in a pot. Add 500ml/18fl oz freshly boiled filtered water. Leave to steep for 5–10 minutes, then strain.

There are so many additional or alternative herbs that you could put in this tea. I haven't put them in as they don't taste great, but you might want to give them a go. Motherwort is a potent *nervine* as well as bringing tone and strength to the uterus. It does increase circulation in the pelvis though, so don't use it if you have heavy bleeding. Another herb useful for balancing the cycle is vitex agnus-castus (chasteberry). It is useful where there is a feeling of liverishness before the period due to a lack of progesterone. It is best taken as a tincture with the guidance of a herbalist.

Chamomile flower This yellow flower is a potent protector of health. It can balance oestrogen levels as well as reduce any inflammation that may lead to menstrual spasms and pain. Its gentle effect on digestion will help you metabolise your hormones and optimise nutrition by making your digestive system work better.

Shatavari root This sweet root is a part of the juicy asparagus family. It is a wonderful women's tonic that can help to nourish oestrogen levels and build energy where there may be fatigue. It's especially helpful for women with short or irregular cycles.

Hibiscus flower The beautiful rosy red hibiscus is refreshingly sour and famed for nourishing the blood. As the health of the blood is so obviously connected with a healthy menstrual cycle, hibiscus can play a tasty and supportive role here.

Dandelion root A very reliable bittersweet liver tonic that helps metabolise your hormones. It also eases digestion to reduce premenstrual bloating.

Rose flower Soothing to smell and joyous to behold, the rose is a wonderfully calming flower for emotional vagaries that can fluctuate within the monthly cycle. Its astringency also makes it a specific for stopping heavy bleeding.

Licorice root Sweet and strong, licorice softens everything it touches. It has a gentle phyto-oestrogenic effect (it is a plant-based source of natural hormones), and it helps the body to regulate oestrogen by diluting the effects of high oestrogen (if you have too much, it stops the uptake of naturally produced oestrogen) and offsetting the effects of having too little (if you don't have enough, it makes your body think it has more so it behaves in a more healthy balance).

Vanilla pod This delicious fruit pod comes from a member of the exotic orchid family and is a special soothing herb – one smell can harmonise everything from your mood to your digestion.

Man, Woman & Child

This tea celebrates pregnancy and prepares the body for labour. It will bring tone to your uterus and strength to your body. Start drinking it three months before your due date.

Full moon celebrations

Raspberry leaf 4g
Nettle leaf 4g
Shatavari root 2g
Fennel seed 1g
Peppermint leaf 1g

This will serve 2–3 cups of perfect partum-preparation tea.

Put all of the ingredients in a pot. Add 500ml/18fl oz freshly boiled filtered water. Leave to steep for 5–10 minutes, then strain.

Raspberry leaf Long used as a support during the last months of pregnancy, raspberry leaf helps ease both the effort and duration of labour. Not as tasty as the berries, it has a very mild herby flavour that is slightly astringent. It helps to tonify the uterus and bring strength to its smooth muscles.

Nettle leaf If it isn't already, nettle leaf becomes a great friend of every expectant mother-in-the-know by month six. Its nutrient-rich content (including Vitamin B, C, K, beta-carotene, iron, calcium, magnesium, protein and essential fatty acids) brings strength to you and your baby.

Shatavari root Ayurveda's favourite herb for rejuvenating women's health, shatavari excels at this stage of pregnancy. Its strengthening properties help you thrive during the final phase of pregnancy and prepares you for the next phase of motherhood by strengthening your blood and giving you more energy.

Fennel seed Good for the digestive system, fennel helps with discomfort that can happen as your baby takes up your tummy's space.

Peppermint leaf Soothing all spasms, peppermint brings relaxation to your digestion.

See a herbalist or doctor if you need any specific pregnancy advice.

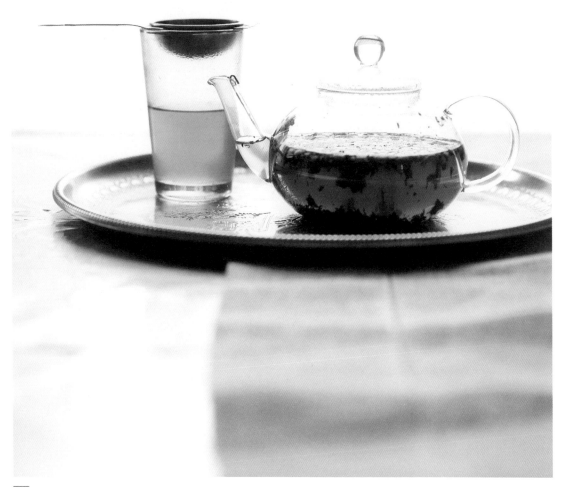

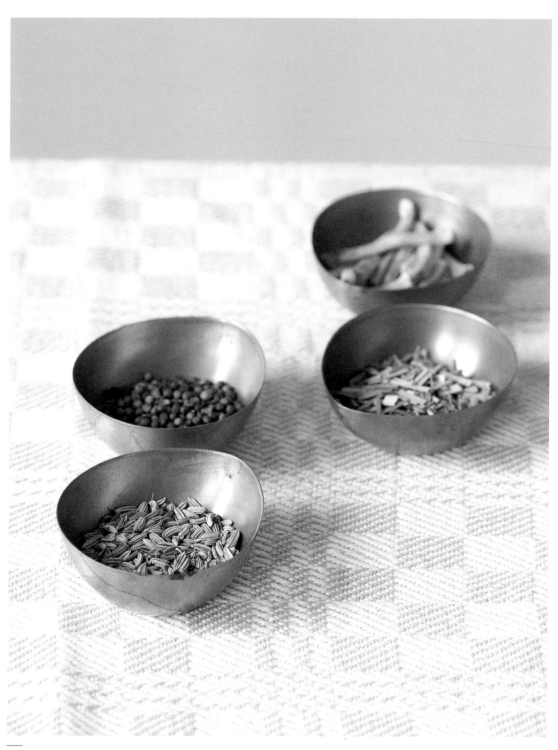

Mother's milk

This is food for mother and child. The herbs in this blend help breast milk flow more freely. About 15 per cent of new mothers experience some form of insufficient milk supply, and this tea will help you avoid being one of them.

Shatavari root 4g
Fennel seed 2g
Coriander seed 2g
Lemongrass leaf 2g

This will serve 2–3 cups of tea that will help your milk flow.

Put all of the ingredients in a pot. Add 500ml/18fl oz freshly boiled filtered water. Leave to steep for 5–10 minutes, then strain.

Shatavari root Famed as a women's rejuvenative fertility tonic, shatavari is a fantastic herb to take after delivery to help support a new mother's strength as well as the flow of breast milk.

Fennel seed A valuable *galactagogue* (helps breast milk flow) that regulates hormones. Known in Ayurveda as *madhurika*, meaning 'the sweet one', fennel balances all three constitutional *dosha*s to restore harmony to the whole system.

Coriander seed Shimmering with essential oils that encourage relaxation and an easy flow of breast milk.

Lemongrass leaf This citrus leaf is full of essential oils that help relax and open our pores, easing the flow of milk and making it taste tempting.

Also think about making and drinking Golden Milk of Bliss on p73 to keep you strong. For an extra boost, add 2g Shatavari root to the recipe.

Man, Woman & Child

The herbs in this blend help you find balance during menopausal change by regulating fluctuating hormones, reducing hot flushes and helping you find your new centre. Yes, a tea *can* cool you down, and this one can definitely ease you through this time of transition.

Cool lady

Sage leaf 3g
Shatavari root 2g
Red clover 2g
Passion flower 2g
Chamomile flower 2g
Fennel seed 1g
Licorice root 1g

This will serve 2–3 cups of cool tea.

Put all of the ingredients in a pot. Add 500ml/18fl oz freshly boiled filtered water. Leave to steep for 10–15 minutes, then strain. Drink it when it's reasonably cool.

Sage leaf A naturally supportive herb, in the sense that it 'holds' things in place. It helps to centre your awareness in the heart, subtly recalibrating your focus until it is one-pointed. This holding effect is what helps sage stop you sweating and keep you grounded during hot flushes and night sweats. It also holds memory in place and is taken by our elders to sustain and support their 'sage-ness'.

Shatavari root A cooling, lubricating and strengthening root, which helps to balance the hot, dry and draining symptoms that can appear at this time of life. It powerfully protects the deeper tissues, bones, nerves and libido.

Red clover As its folklore name 'bee bread' implies, red clover is a life-sustaining food. Its pink clusters of beauty support the hormonal shift by bringing cooling sustenance to your cells. A respected protector of breast and ovarian health, red clover has a special affinity for clearing inflammation from the blood and lymphatic system.

Passion flower Nothing to do with amorous desire, its name dates back to the 15th and 16th centuries when missionaries adopted this resplendent flower as a symbol of the Passion of Christ. It's a climber plant, and this nature is reflected in its journey through the body's nervous system to the crown of the head. On arrival it quickly calms the mind, stills all thoughts and puts your brain in crystal-clear mode. It's in this tea because it's especially useful for menopausal anxiety and insomnia.

Chamomile flower Chamomile works in harmony with the passion flower, helping to manage mood swings and a busy brain. Its eye-like delicate flowers help us to 'see' life through a new lens, one that is much calmer as though our peripheral vision has just widened.

Continued overleaf

Man, Woman & Child

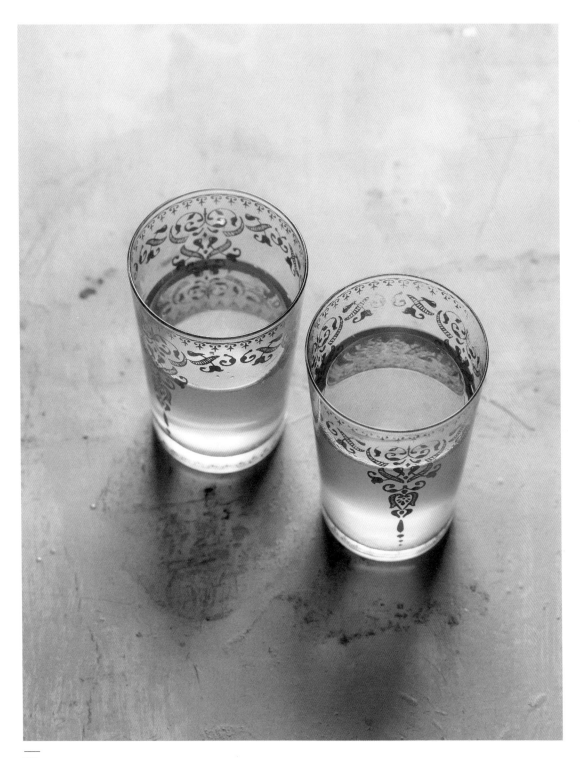

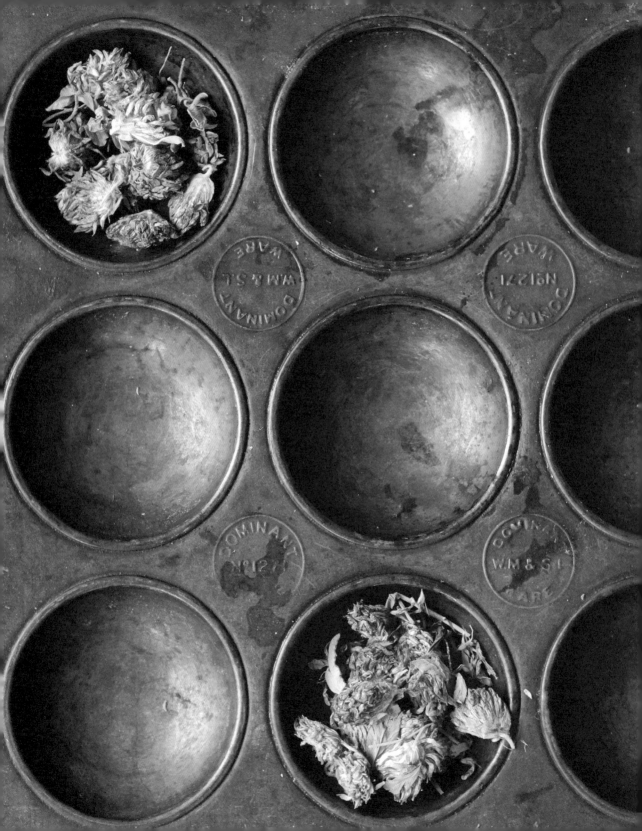

Cool lady

Fennel seed It contains essential oil compounds that help the body to produce oestrogen. Fennel seed calms the system, soothes digestion, helps with menstrual irregularity and reminds you that life tastes good.

Licorice root In its natural habitat, licorice root copes with heat and dryness and its roots burrow down many metres. Reflected in its action in the body, it can cool and moisten, as well as help you feel grounded in the face of change.

Man, Woman & Child

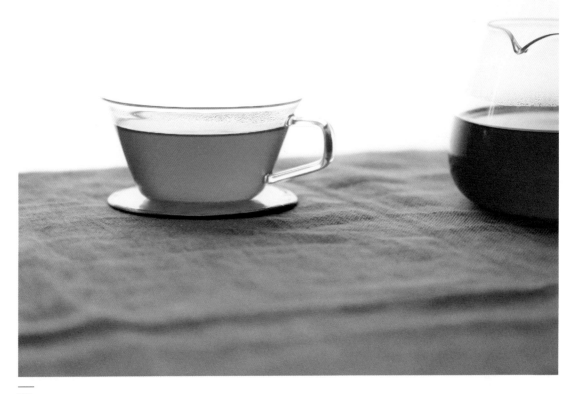

It is common to have painful periods, but it shouldn't be the norm. At some stage, most women experience them. Discovered by wisewomen, midwives and our herbalist ancestors, the herbs in this tea offer a solution: they quicken the blood, relax spasms and help your life-force flow more freely as they remove the root of the discomfort.

Monthly liberation

Cramp bark 5g
Fennel seed 4g
Turmeric root powder 3g
Valerian root 2g
Ginger root powder 1g

This will serve 2–3 cups of liberating pain relief tea.

Put all of the ingredients in a pot. Add 500ml/18fl oz freshly boiled filtered water. Leave to steep for 15 minutes, then strain. To make a stronger brew for a bolder effect, put the herbs in a pan and cover with a lid. Bring to the boil and allow to simmer for 15 minutes, then strain.

Sit with a hot water bottle on your belly while you drink this one. If you have got the blues, make a cup of Let There By Joy on p116 , too.

Cramp bark The name says it all. It is specific for calming uterine spasms which cause period pains. It also helps relax muscles, reduces lower back pain and eases the dragging-into-the-thighs sensation that can be so uncomfortable.

Fennel seed Fennel has a long history of helping the menses flow and is a specific for period pain. It relaxes tension, eases spasms and lets your energy flow. It also helps with any tummy upset or nausea that can occur from the pain.

Turmeric root Also known as the Golden Goddess in India, turmeric root thins the blood, helping it move more easily. It also works just like a pharmaceutical painkiller as it inhibits inflammatory pathways in the body (such as the cyclooxygenase pathway). It stops an enxyme called Substance-P sending messages of pain to our brain. Turmeric is one of nature's best painkillers.

Valerian root A marvellous quick-acting pain reliever, valerian root goes straight into your nervous system, freeing you from spasms, cramps and pain. It's warming, moving and grounding. Valerian root does have a rather strong smell.

Ginger root Warming and invigorating, ginger quickens the flow of blood through the uterus, which gets a slow-moving period going and swiftly removes any pain. Think of ginger whenever there is a delayed, scanty, painful or clotty period. Its also a fine antispasmodic and anti-inflammatory.

Man, Woman & Child

Little one's calm cup

Our wild and wonderful world can be overwhelming at times. Whether it's growing so quickly, learning so much every day or just being in a whirl of change, it can all easily mount up and make children feel tense. As you would expect, mother nature is close at hand to help with some super-soothing herbs.

Limeflower 2g
Lemon balm 2g
Chamomile flower 2g
Honey to taste

This will serve 2–3 cups of cooling calmness. For more on dosages for children, see p161 and p25.

Put all of the ingredients in a pot. Add 500ml/18fl oz freshly boiled filtered water. Leave to steep for 5–10 minutes, then strain and let it cool. Add a touch of honey for some sweetness.

Limeflower Also known as linden, this fragrant blossom is heaven in a cup. Its soft, sweet, silky experience takes the hard edges off everything. It cools irritability, encourages patience and soothes a furrowed brow.

Lemon balm The light, ethereal quality of lemon balm helps you see the calm in the eye of the storm. It stems anxiety by encouraging security and confidence when the unconscious fear of failure and low self-esteem loom.

Chamomile flower Surviving in the tough wilds, chamomile helps the oversensitive build protection. Its gentle and loving nature brings a sense of peace when feeling unsettled and will help little ones feel more relaxed and calm.

Turn to this tea if your little one is tense, anxious, restless or sleepless.

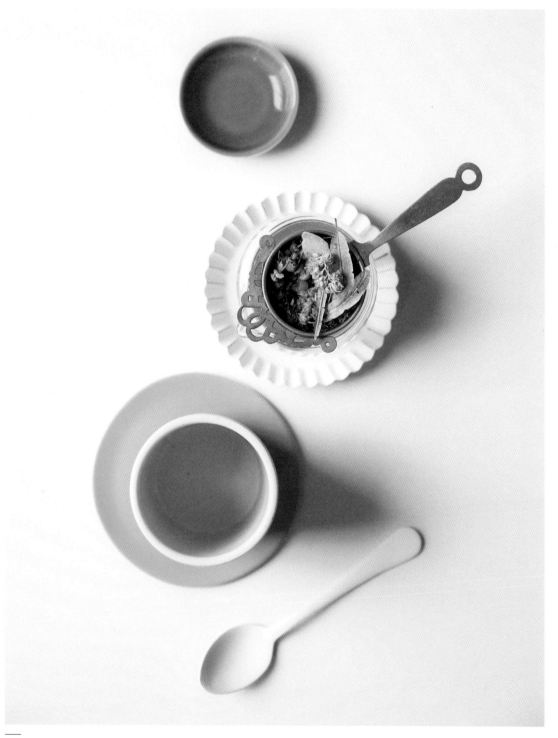

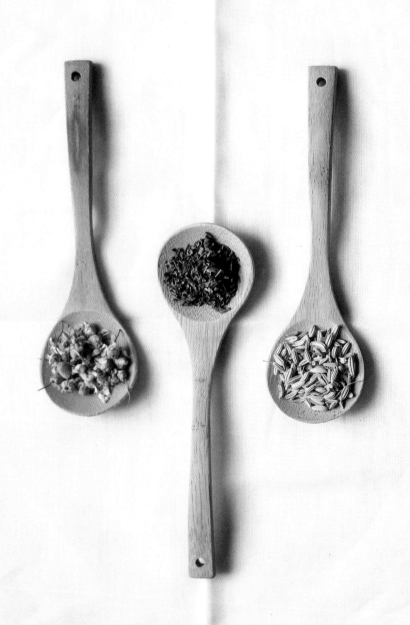

A child's digestive system faces a double challenge: it has to manage the constant demands of food while also maturing and growing. This can lead to erratic eating and tummy upsets.

Little one's tummy tea

Fennel seed 2g
Peppermint leaf 2g
Chamomile flower 2g
Honey to taste

This will serve 2–3 cups of tummy-calming bliss. For more on dosages for children, see p161 and p25.

Put all of the ingredients in a pot. Add 500ml/18fl oz freshly boiled filtered water. Leave to steep for 5–10 minutes, then strain and let it cool. Add a touch of honey for some sweetness.

Use this tea as a simple aid to digestion after a meal. Many children's health issues start in the digestive system, and this tea will help it (and them) stay strong.

Fennel seed Children love the flavour and the feeling of fennel's sweet seed. Its essential oils gently percolate into the tea and soothe a belly-ache with just a few sips. It strengthens the digestive fire so children can absorb their food better.

Peppermint leaf Delightful mint assists a struggling digestion and calms nausea, gas and griping. As you breathe mint in, you can feel it having an opening effect – it also has this effect in your tummy.

Chamomile flower Soothing chamomile brings calm and reduces tension in griping tummies. The essential oils work synergistically to stop spasms and help absorption of nutrients. Many clinical trials have shown how chamomile can bring relief to little ones with colic.

Little one's cold tea

When children overload their digestive system it can cause mucus to brim over. Infectious microbes that land on that 'sludge' have a welcome home to proliferate and lead to the ubiquitous runny nose and chesty cough that children so often suffer from. As well as this tea, lighten their diet and let them take rest.

Catnip leaf 2g
Chamomile flower 2g
Elderflower 1g
Fresh ginger root 1 slice
Honey to taste

This will serve 2–3 cups of get-me-better-quickly tea. For more on dosages for children, see p161 and p25.

Put all of the ingredients in a pot. Add 500ml/18fl oz freshly boiled filtered water. Leave to steep for 5–10 minutes, then strain and let it cool. Add a touch of honey for some sweetness.

Catnip leaf Catnip is a member of the mint family and has similar dispersing and opening effects – it disperses a stuffy chest and opens a blocked nose. It's a traditional favourite for cooling children's fevers as it's quick to act and tastes good. It can increase circulation, which diffuses feverish heat.

Chamomile flower The children's panacea, chamomile relaxes the tension brought on by feeling ill, while also clearing the chest of mucus.

Elderflower A specific for chesty coughs that linger in the winter damp, elderflower raises energy and immunity alike.

Ginger root A little warmth pushes the cold up and out. Ginger's stimulating effect on the lungs clears the mucus and dries out the damp where needed (lungs, digestive system, urinary system).

If your little one gets recurring colds, give them a warm elderberry drink as well. See Elderberry Elixir on p144.

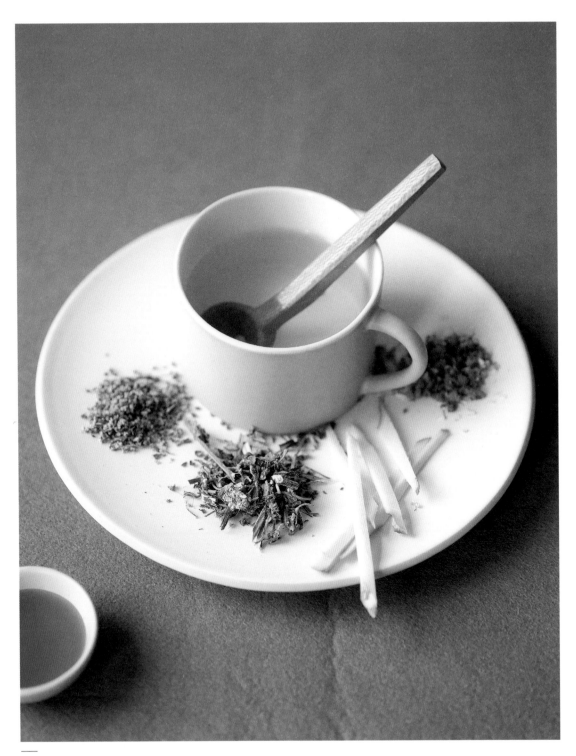

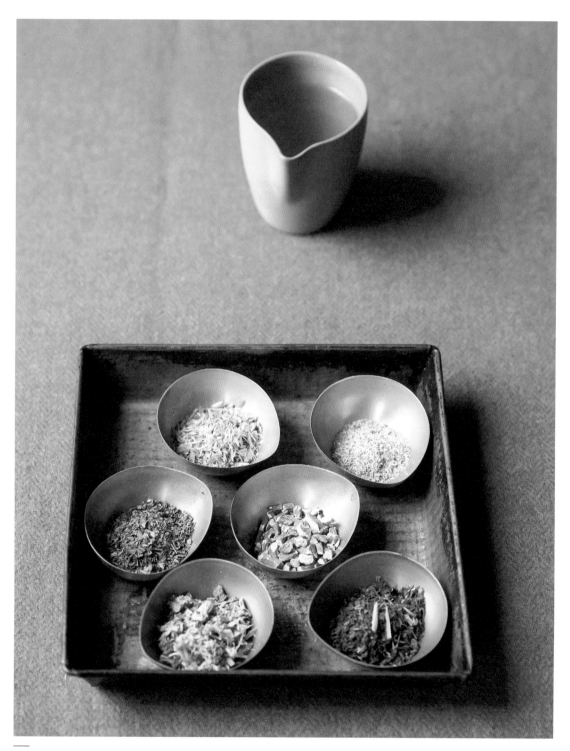

Becoming a teenager is as wonderful as it is bizarre. Growing into yourself is something that we do forever, but the change is most stark as we enter puberty. Growing self-awareness is usually blended with a mix of excitement and awe as we begin to realise our power and the opportunities and responsibilities that go with it. Drink this tea to keep you cool as you work your way through school. It will help keep your skin glowing, hormones balanced and mood bright.

Too cool for school

Oat straw flowering top 4g
Nettle leaf 2g
Peppermint leaf 1g
Dandelion root 1g
Burdock root 1g
Licorice root 1g
Honey to taste

This will serve 2–3 cups of tip-top-teen tea.

Put all of the ingredients in a pot. Add 500ml/18fl oz freshly boiled filtered water. Leave to steep for 5–10 minutes, then strain and let it cool. Add a touch of honey for some sweetness.

Oat straw flowering top A gentle nervous system restorative that promotes balance in the face of change. Think of oat straw as a tonic for making you strong physically and emotionally.
Nettle leaf Its nutrient profile (Vitamin B, C, K, beta-carotene, iron, calcium, magnesium, protein and essential fatty acids) helps us manage change by building our strength so that we are more robust in the face of transformation.
Peppermint leaf Very useful for digesting voluminous plates of pasta, pizza, chocolate and all things heavy, greasy and sweet.
Dandelion root Adolescence brings a wellspring of ardent passion and heat. This can overflow into your skin, causing acne that dandelion can help to wash away.
Burdock root The idea for making Velcro came from the sticky burr on burdock seed – and aptly the burdock root catches all of our sticky mess and takes it away (think toxins – often from a junk food diet – that lead to spots). It is known as an *alterative* that helps alter our inner chemistry and moves us towards health. It's especially good for cleansing the skin and keeping it clear of teenage acne.
Licorice root The sweetness of licorice sends a message to your brain that everything is alright, and so your brain sends balancing messages back to our body. Everything is cool.

Man, Woman & Child

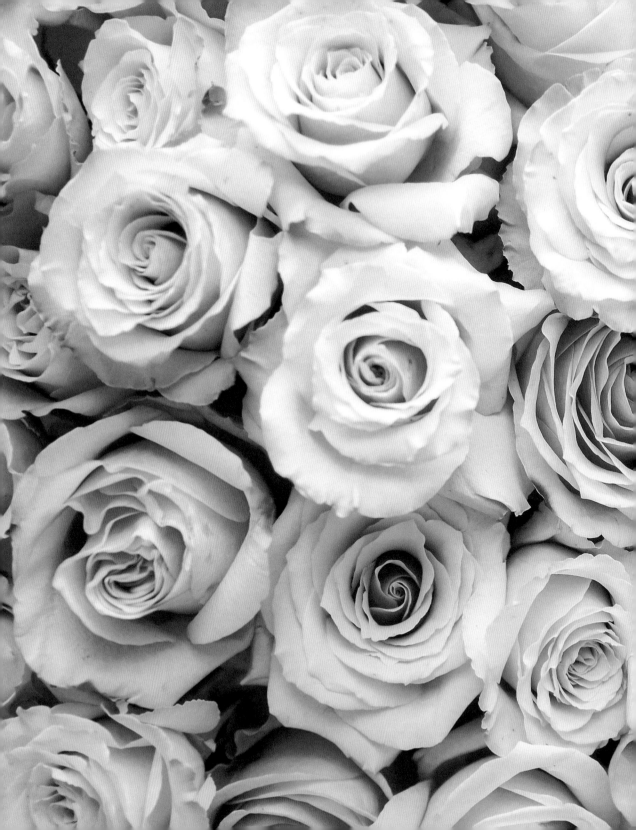

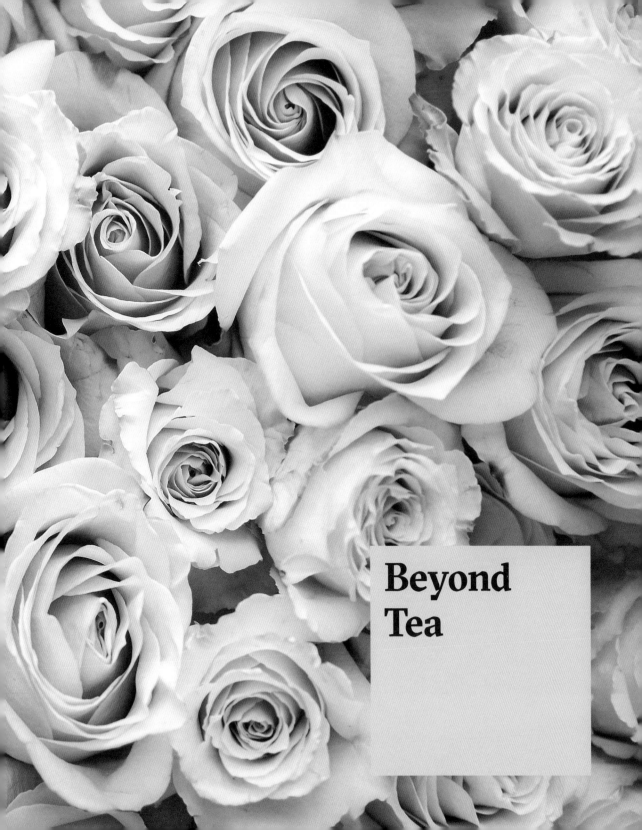

Beyond Tea

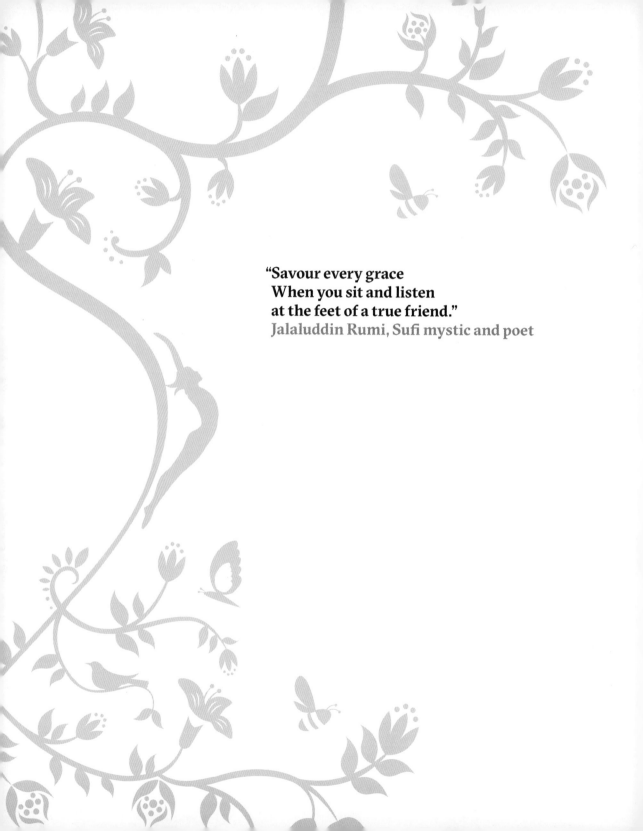

"Savour every grace
 When you sit and listen
 at the feet of a true friend."
Jalaluddin Rumi, Sufi mystic and poet

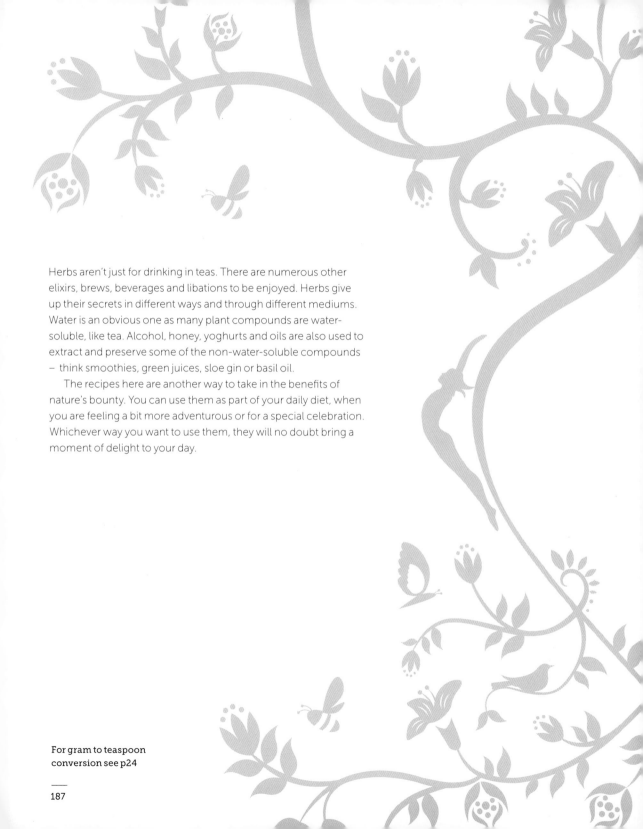

Herbs aren't just for drinking in teas. There are numerous other elixirs, brews, beverages and libations to be enjoyed. Herbs give up their secrets in different ways and through different mediums. Water is an obvious one as many plant compounds are water-soluble, like tea. Alcohol, honey, yoghurts and oils are also used to extract and preserve some of the non-water-soluble compounds – think smoothies, green juices, sloe gin or basil oil.

The recipes here are another way to take in the benefits of nature's bounty. You can use them as part of your daily diet, when you are feeling a bit more adventurous or for a special celebration. Whichever way you want to use them, they will no doubt bring a moment of delight to your day.

For gram to teaspoon conversion see p24

A lassi is a traditional Indian drink made with yoghurt, water and various other delights. It is one of the most delicious drinks you'll ever make.

Rose essence lassi

Fresh rose syrup
Fresh organic rose petal
   2 large handfuls
Honey 300g/10oz

Rose water syrup
Rose water 150ml/5fl oz
Honey 300g/10oz

For the lassi
Yoghurt 100g/4oz
Filtered water 100ml/3⅓fl oz
Fresh rose syrup 1 tbsp
   (or rose water syrup 1 tbsp)

This will serve 1 cup of lovely lassi.

Blend the yoghurt with the water, then add the rose syrup. With each sip the roses help you to open your heart and taste joy.

Yoghurt Warming, wet and heavy with a sweet-sour taste, yoghurt has plenty to recommend it. In Ayurveda, it reduces dry-*vata* and increases hot-*pitta* and damp-*kapha*. It benefits digestion, nourishes fertility and cures diarrhoea. According to Ayurveda, it should never be eaten at night, in the winter or in very hot summers cold from the fridge, or without mixing it with spices, ghee, honey, sugar, mung beans or amla fruit. This is because it has a unique negative property that obstructs the flow of the water element in the body and blocks the channels of circulation. This hydrophilic property leads to mucus build-up, fluid retention and congestion. If you'd like to get the best from your yoghurt, dilute it with water and add digestive spices (such as cumin, ginger or coriander) to turn it into a healing elixir.

To make the fresh rose syrup
Add the fresh organic rose petals to a bowl and cover with the honey. Leave overnight. In the morning, strain the liquid off through a fine sieve. Store the syrup in the fridge.

To make the rose water syrup
Add the rose water and honey to a bottle and shake until the honey has dissolved into the rose water. Store the syrup in the fridge.

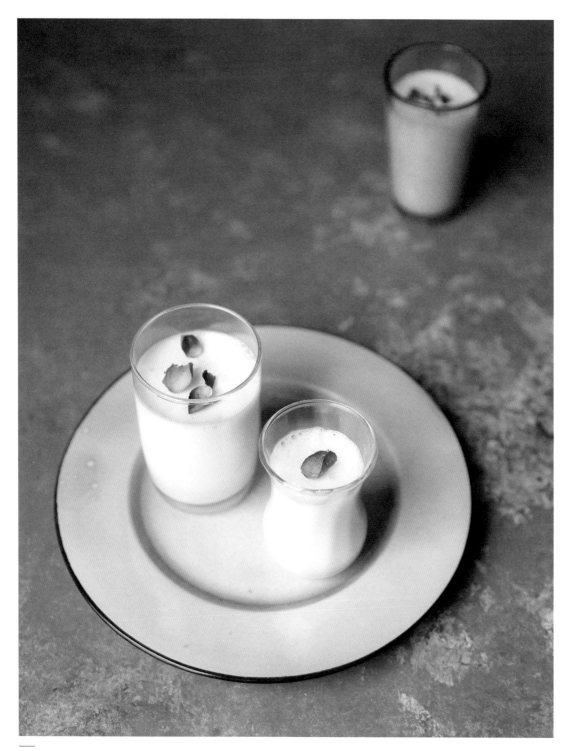

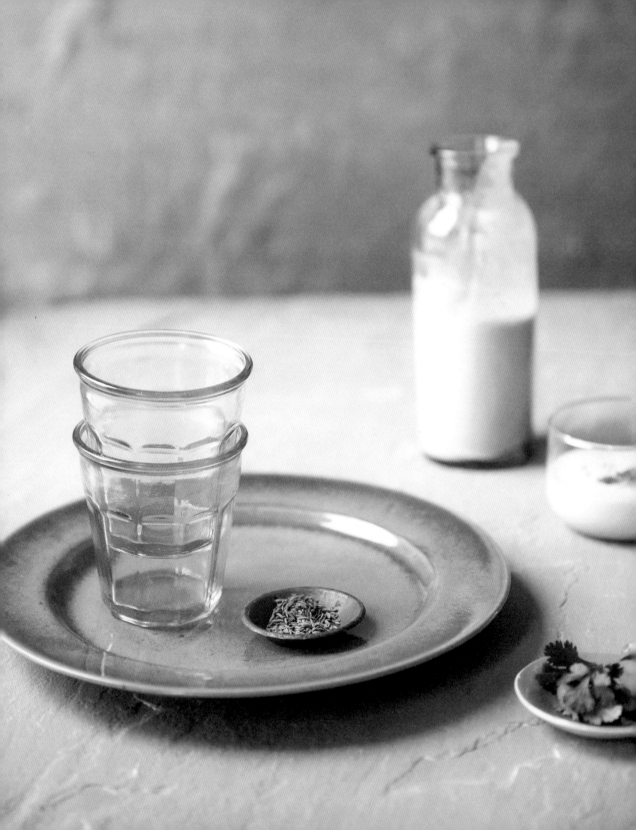

Digestive lassi

This is a favourite digestive drink recommended in Ayurveda to increase the digestive fire and help digestion. Great with a meal.

Fresh coriander 10g, about 1 handful
Fresh ginger root 2 slices
Ground cumin a pinch
Salt a pinch
Yoghurt 100g/4oz
Filtered water 100ml/3½fl oz

This will serve 1 cup of digestion-fuelling drink.

Finely chop the fresh coriander and ginger. Blend the yoghurt with the water. Add the fresh herbs with a pinch of cumin and salt. Blend again and enjoy.

This is a wonderful drink for supporting the digestion. It helps build your gut flora (the microorganisms in the digestive tract), aids in the assimilation of nutrients and assists in settling your digestion after a meal. The fresh ginger, cumin and salt are stimulating to digestion, while the fresh coriander is full of aromatic essential oils that help to support digestion.

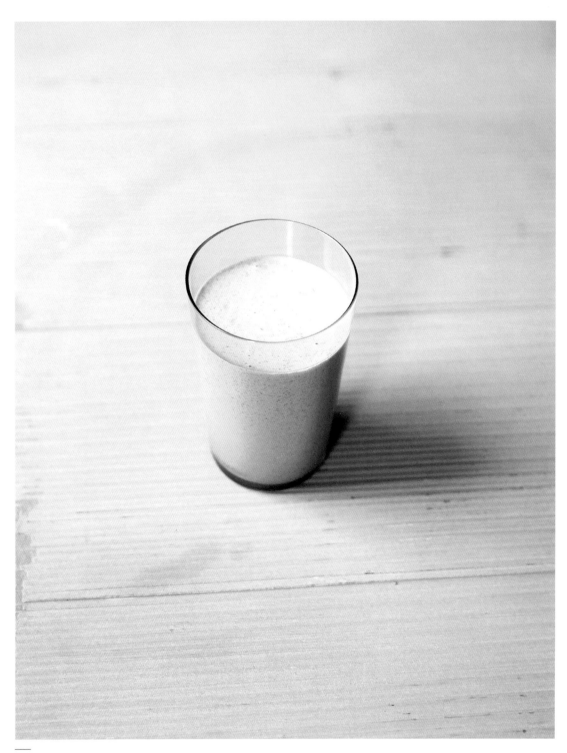

The seeds of life

An excellent way to get a source of easy-to-digest protein and healthy fats. This rich elixir gets you off to a flying start.

Coconut yoghurt 100g/4oz
Coconut oil 1 tbsp
Almond (or other) milk 150ml/5¼fl oz
   (you can use the almond milk recipe
   on p70: follow the method but exclude
   the saffron, cardamom and honey)
Pumpkin seed 1 tbsp
Walnuts 1 tbsp
Linseed 1 tbsp
Hemp seed oil 2 tbsp
Ground fennel seed a pinch
Ground cardamom a pinch

This will serve 1 cup of good-life.

Soak the pumpkin seeds, walnuts and linseeds in a cup of water overnight to get them sprouting with life. Then drain them the next morning and blend together with the rest of the ingredients. This one keeps you going.

Fat is good for you. That is a fact. Our body absolutely requires us to eat good quality fat in our diet in order to process such fat-soluble nutrients such as Vitamins A, D, E and K as well as to absorb protective phytochemicals (such as the colourful flavonoids and carotenoids) and certain minerals. It is essential for creating enough digestive enzymes. We need it to regulate hormone production, it gives us energy, it helps regulate our moods, it protects our organs and it keeps us warm. Our brains are 60 per cent fat and we have around 15kg/33lbs of it in our body. Our nervous system, our brains, our eyes, our joints are all comprised in part from fat. When thinking about whether fat is good or bad, as with all Ayurvedic principles, it comes down to how much of what is consumed by whom and when.

Essential fatty acids (also known as omega oils) are as essential to life as vitamins and minerals. And because we can't make them ourselves we have to get them from our diet. Both omega-6 (linoleic acid) and omega-3 (alpha linolenic acid) essential fatty acids are important building blocks in the body's metabolism and building of our precious cellular membranes. In general, omega-6 fats tend to promote inflammation, constriction of the blood vessels and formation of blood cell clots. Omega-3 fats have the opposite effect: they're anti-inflammatory, relax the blood vessels, lower blood pressure and protect against blood cells aggregating together into clots.

Hemp seed contains the highest amount of essential fatty acids of any vegetable oil (80 per cent). The EFAs in hemp seed oil include omega-6, omega-3 and GLA (gamma linolenic acid). GLA is a rare nutrient found in mother's milk. Hemp seed oil has a ratio of omega-6 to omega-3 of 3:1, and this is nature's natural range for the most perfect balance for optimum health.

Continued overleaf

The seeds of life

Women need 3 tablespoons and men 4 tablespoons a day of hemp seed oil to get suitable levels of EPA and DHA. Women need less but convert it better.

In terms of healthy fats, virgin coconut oil is easily digestible and contains medium chain triglycerides/fatty acids (MCTs), which increase the metabolic rate, impacting directly upon the efficiency of the digestive system and the liver. Virgin coconut oil does not require the pancreatic fat-digesting enzyme lipase in order to be digested, and goes straight to the liver to be transformed into energy. This bypasses the usual fat digestion journey, reducing the risk of imbalanced cholesterol and blood-fat build up. Consequently it can be a healthy addition to balanced weight loss programmes. Its soothing, cooling and oily nature also makes it a perfect remedy for internal and external inflammation and irritation.

Omega-6 is found in sunflower oil, rapeseed oil, corn oil and safflower oils; processed foods are often high in these oils.

Omega-3 is found in hemp seed oil, flax seed oil, walnut oil and pumpkin seed oil. (Also some fish like salmon and tuna but they don't taste good in a smoothie.)

While omega-6 fatty acids are necessary for normal immune function and clotting, too much omega-6 fatty acid may promote abnormal clotting and an imbalanced immune system. It is believed that our ancestors evolved on a diet where these two omega fatty acids were approximately equal. However, modern diets usually have up to 20 times more omega-6 than omega-3 fatty acids. Many of our chronic degenerative diseases today are believed to have their origins in an imbalance of omega-3 and omega-6 fatty acids in our diet. This necessitates that they be consumed in a balanced proportion. Healthy ratios of omegas-6 to 3 range from 1:1 to 4:1. And this is where the seeds of life come in.

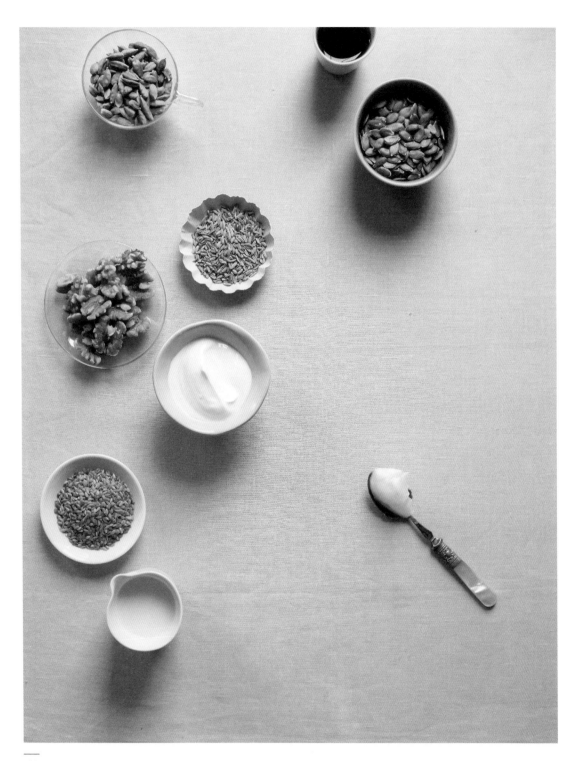

This drink helps you to feel clean instantly. But taken over a few weeks its chlorophyll and minerals can really help alkalise, wash and restore your tissues. It's good for your skin, eyes, blood and it boosts your vitamin, mineral and phytonutrient levels.

Clean greens

Wheatgrass juice, powder or
   Pukka Clean Greens powder
   1 tsp
Avocado 1 (peeled and pitted)
Cucumber ¼ stick
Celery 1 stick
Green leaves (such as spinach
   rocket/kale) 2 large handfuls
Fresh mint leaves 6
Fresh coriander 10g (about
   1 handful)
Lemon juice ½ a lemon
Black pepper a pinch
Fresh ginger root 2cm/¾in
Fresh turmeric root 2cm/¾in
Aloe vera juice 1 tbsp
Himalayan rock salt a pinch
Dried seaweed ½ tsp
300ml/10½fl oz filtered water

This will serve 2 cups of goodness-boosting drink.

Place all the ingredients into a blender and whizz until smooth. Enjoy while it's fresh.

Chlorophyll captures the sun's energy and transforms it so that life can flourish on earth. The only difference between chlorophyll and haem (the oxygen-carrying portion of haemoglobin) molecules is the magnesium at the centre of chlorophyll and the iron at the centre of haemoglobin. This could be one of the reasons why chlorophyll can be of such benefit to the blood. It has the ability to cleanse while re-building at the same time. This makes it the perfect solution to keep you fresh and energised. Mixed with a plethora of beneficial nutrients, chlorophyll carries its cooling and calming properties deep into the tissues. The chlorophyll in these greens has the ability to nourish red blood cells and is therefore helpful in blood deficient anaemia as well as inflammation in the digestive system (and elsewhere).

Wheatgrass juice contains a plethora of bio-active nutrients and enzymes, which are naturally occurring proteins that act as catalysts to metabolic activity, specifically supporting immune function, elimination of free radicals, detoxification and energy production. Wheatgrass juice is famed for inducing a rapid healing response due to its high levels of detoxifying glutathione. It is also rich in superoxide dismutase, one of the most prominent bio-active enzymes, which helps to generate glutathione and slow cellular degeneration, ageing and general wrinkling.

Seaweed is nourishing and detoxifying. It cleanses the lymph, benefits the thyroid and assists with weight loss. It's steeped in all the trace minerals of the land that have washed into the sea over millennia.

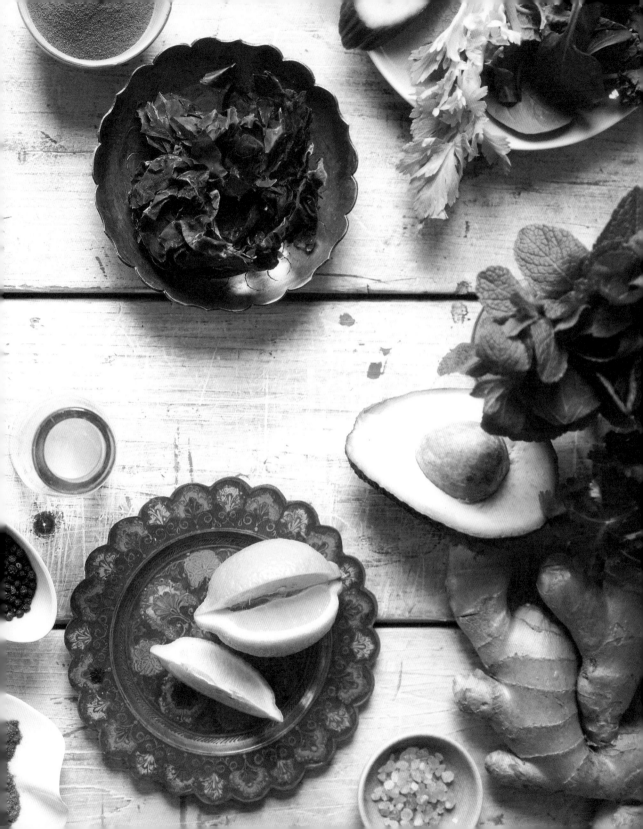

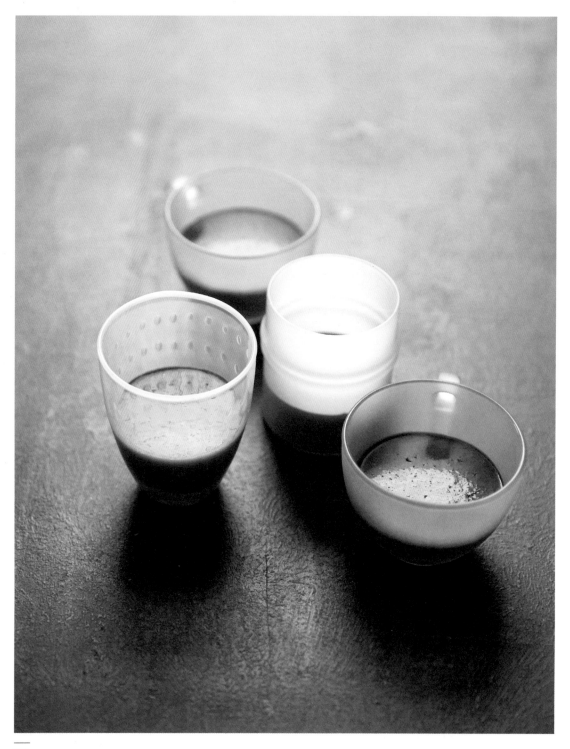

Drink this gloriously coloured super booster as a nourishing and revitalising energy tonic that is glowing with vitamins, minerals and antioxidants.

Vitalise berry boost

Berries (any blue, black, red or purple ones) 100g/4oz, about 1 handful
A red superfood supplement like Pukka's Vitalise 1 tbsp
Pomegranate juice 200ml/7fl oz
Hemp seed oil 1 tbsp
Amla powder 1 tsp
Honey to taste (optional)

This will serve 2 cups of goodness-boosting drink.

Blend all the ingredients together with a touch of water until smooth.

Berries, such as acerola, amla, blueberries, bilberries, blackberries, blackcurrants and elderberries are packed with vitamins and phytonutrients (the flavonoids quercetin, ellagic acid and phenolic compounds like resveratrol, anthocyanins and proanthocyanins – anthocyanins are what give the fruits their characteristic red, blue and purple vibrancy). Berries have renowned anti-ageing and antioxidant benefits, as they help to protect our cells from oxidation. They help by protecting us from absorbing harmful oxidative products that can damage the DNA through something called the 'lipo-peroxidising effect'. They protect the precious lipids in the cell membrane, slow the reproduction of rogue cells, and immobilise mutated cells. This helps us to age gracefully and healthily. Their juices stop the blood forming clots by reducing platelet levels, giving circulatory system support and benefits to those at risk from strokes and heart attacks. They also reduce inflammation and strengthen the body's collagen tissue.

The amla fruit, also known as Indian gooseberry, rejuvenates all three *dosha*s and is best used to remove fatigue from the body. Amla's hallmark as a great healer is its therapeutic flexibility: it is an immune stimulant (beneficial for short-term infections) and also an *adaptogen* that deeply nourishes immunity to offer long-term protection from degenerative disease. Its powerful antioxidant capacity can help delay ageing and prolong life and is useful whenever there is chronic inflammation and/or weakness in the digestive system, liver, blood or heart. It is a part of the famous Triphala formula and one of Ayurveda's most important remedies. It is also one of the main ingredients in chyawanprash (the nutritious Ayurvedic jam), which is another good way to get your daily dose of amla.

This is a fun and easy-to-make elixir. It will set you on the path of herbal experimentation as you can use the principle of this recipe with any alcohol that is more than 25 per cent proof together with any herbs. Make this as the nights start to draw in for warming your winter evenings.

Winter tonic elixir

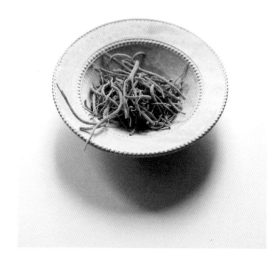

Brandy 700ml/25fl oz
Amaretto 300ml/10fl oz
Ginseng root 20g/¾oz
Astragalus 10g/⅓oz
Cinnamon bark 10g (about 2 quills)
Ashwagandha 5g
Ginger root powder 5g
Rosemary 2 sprigs
Orange peel 5g

This makes 1 litre/35fl oz of tasty tincture.

Blend the liquids and soak the herbs in the blend for 1 month. Strain, then bottle half for you and half for a friend. Sip on cold winter nights to raise your spirits and keep you strong.

These herbs are all rejuvenating tonics that raise your energy, lift your life-force and warm you to your core. Ginseng, astragalus and ashwagandha build deep energy, while cinnamon, ginger and rosemary invigorate your circulation and warm you from the top of your head to the tips of your toes.

Make this wild-foraged potion to support your immunity through the winter. Gathering the berries and fruits is a way of capturing some of nature's most protective herbs as they help to ward off colds.

Fruits of the forest

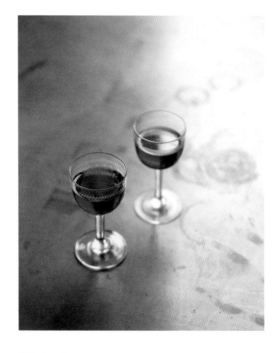

Fresh elderberry 60g/2oz
Fresh hawthorn berry 30g/1oz
Rosehip 60g/2oz
Fresh raspberry 60g/2oz
Fresh sloe berry 30g/1oz
Vodka (40% abv/80 proof) 700ml/25fl oz
Honey 200ml/7fl oz

This makes 1 litre/35fl oz of fruity protector.

Soak the fresh berries in the vodka and honey for a month. Strain, then bottle and enjoy as a winter tonic to ward off the cold and colds.

Elderberries are one of the most potent protectors against respiratory viruses as they actually stop winter lurgies from replicating and spreading. Hawthorn berries are good for your chest and rosehips contain a plethora of protective flavonoids and Vitamin C. Autumn raspberries do a host of things including making this forest elixir taste great.

This drink lets the wild ones sparkle.
Enjoy it with friends.

A supremely wild sparkler

Supreme Matcha Green by Pukka 3 teabags
Three Licorice by Pukka 1 teabag
Fresh mint leaves 1 bunch
Brown sugar 2½ tbsp
White rum 25ml/1 shot per glass
Prosecco (enough to top each glass)

Serves 15 small glasses of sparkle.

Cover the tea bags with 750ml/26fl oz boiled filtered water. Leave to infuse for 20 minutes in a covered container. Strain and cool. Muddle the mint leaves in brown sugar and add one or two leaves to each glass. Fill half of the glass with the tea, add a shot of rum to each glass, then top up with prosecco.

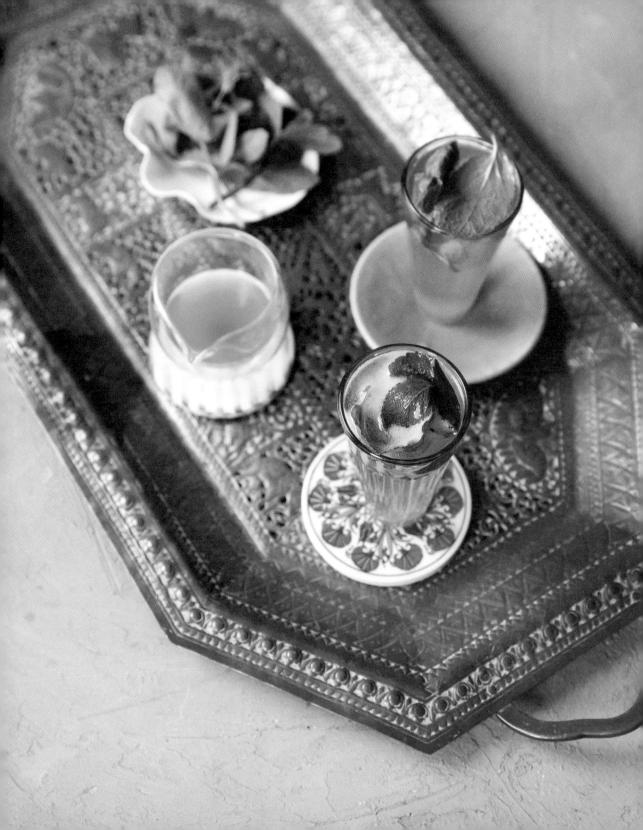

Freshness herself fizzing with the exuberance of life. Make this to bring a little bit of green matcha get-go to your evening.

Three mint matcha mojito

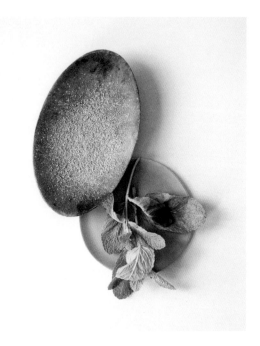

Three Mint by Pukka 3 teabags
Fresh mint 3 leaves per glass
Jaggery (or brown sugar) 1 tbsp
White rum 25ml/1 shot per glass
Lime juice 1 lime
Matcha a sprinkle per glass
Soda water (enough to top each glass)

This will serve 3 cups of fizzy fun.

Cover the teabags with 150ml/5¼fl oz boiling water. Leave to infuse for 30 minutes in a covered container. Strain, then leave to cool in the fridge for 2 hours. Muddle the mint with the sugar. When ready to serve, add to each glass a shot of rum, 2 shots of mint tea and a handful of crushed ice. Add a squeeze of lime, a sprinkle of matcha and a few of the muddled mint leaves. Stir, then top up with soda water.

Beyond Tea

This is glass of pure ginger fun. It's a fabulously spicy drink – perfect for cool summer nights.

The ginger princess

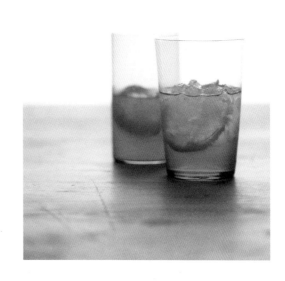

Three Ginger by Pukka 3 teabags
Gin 25ml/1 shot per glass
Lemon juice ¼ lemon
Honey to taste
Ginger ale (enough to top each glass)

This will serve 3 cups of gin and ginger.

Cover the teabags with 150ml/5¼fl oz boiling water. Leave to infuse for 30 minutes in a covered container. Strain, then leave to cool in the fridge for 2 hours. When ready to serve, add to a glass a shot of gin, 2 shots of ginger tea, crushed ice, a twist of lemon and a dash of honey. Stir, then top up with ginger ale.

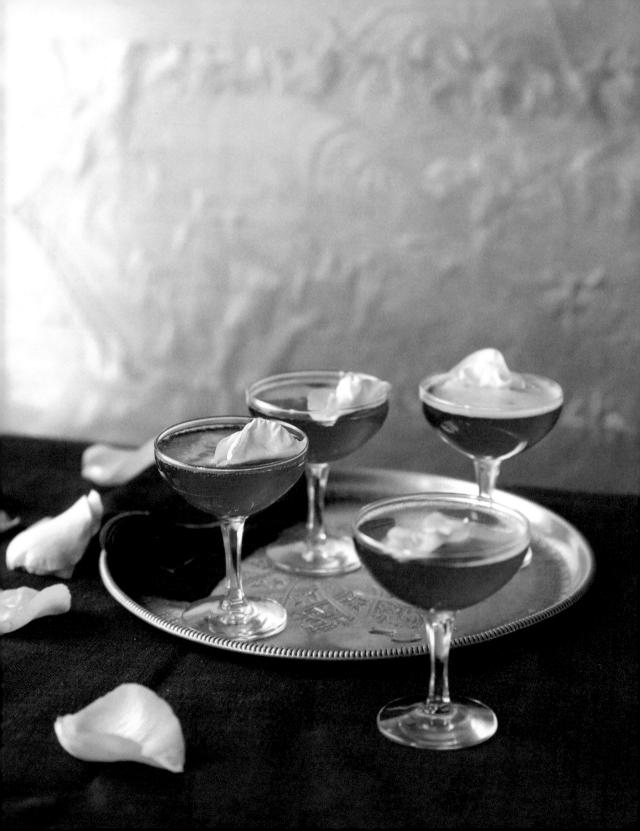

A special drink for special occasions. Whenever we have a party at Pukka I have the pleasurable responsibility of making this cocktail. An original that I made to celebrate our 10th birthday back in 2011, it's since become a classic.

Pukkalini

Love Tea by Pukka 3 teabags
Pomegranate juice 50ml/2 shots per glass
Rose water (optional) 1 tsp per glass
Fresh rose petal (optional) 1 per glass
Champagne (enough to top each glass)

This will serve 3 cups of celebratory fizz.

Cover the teabags with 150ml/5¼fl oz boiling water. Leave to infuse for 30 minutes in a covered container. Strain, then leave to cool in the fridge for 2 hours. When ready to serve, add to a glass 2 shots of Love Tea, 2 shots of pomegranate juice and then top up with champagne. Add some rose water if you would like. Decorate with a fresh rose petal.

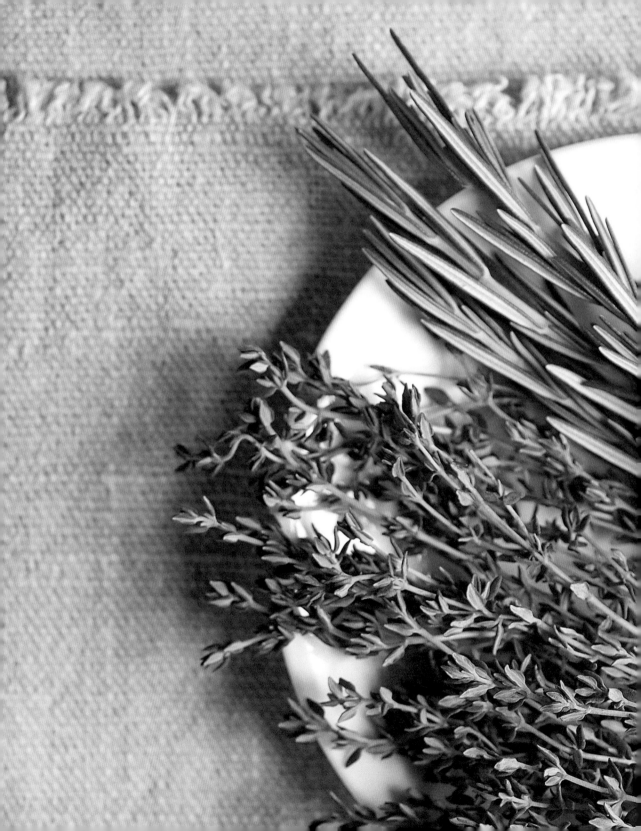

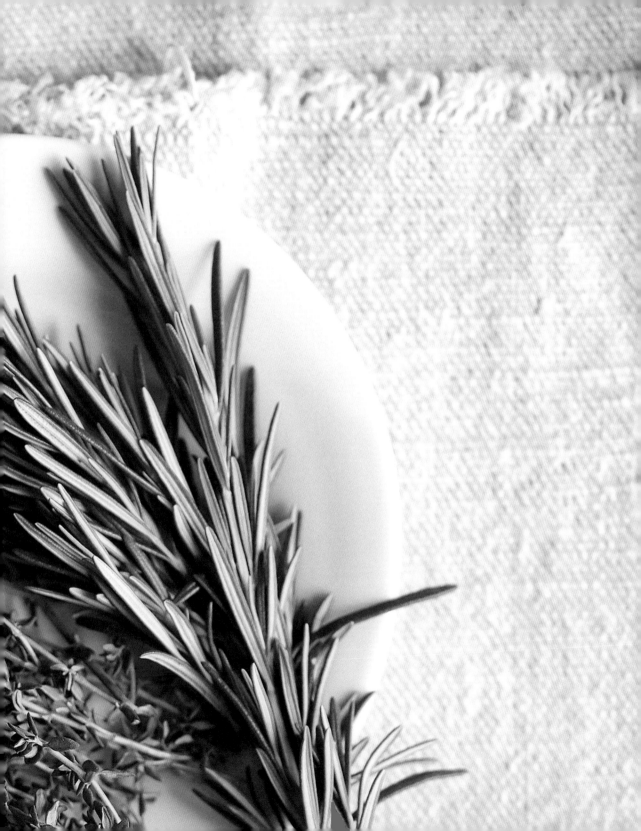

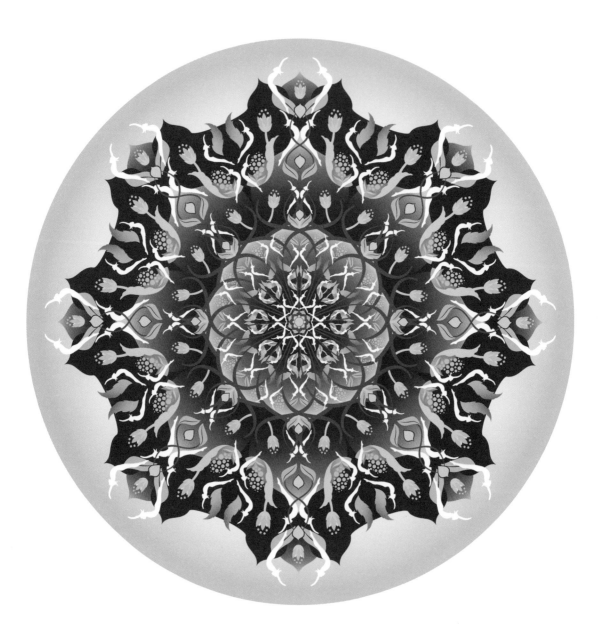

About Ayurveda

Ayurveda is inspiring. It's India's traditional system of holistic health. It describes a way to live that optimises your genetic potential and can transform your life. The essence of Ayurveda fits perfectly with what we want to share at Pukka: we want to connect people to plants and to enhance life's potential.

At its core, Ayurveda teaches respect for nature and an appreciation of life by showing us how we can empower ourselves as individuals. It reminds us that we know the most about ourselves and so in that sense, we can be our own best doctor. The essence of all the food, thoughts and feelings that we bathe our cells in every day become the reality of our health, be it good or bad. Ayurveda's teachings put us in charge of our life, showing us that our environment and our behaviour determine our future.

Ayurveda is a system of medicine and a way of life that adapts with the changes of the seasons, weather, time and place. It teaches dietary and behavioural adjustments that can be adopted as you mature from childhood through to adulthood and into old age. It gives advice on how to prevent illness and specific recommendations on how to fine-tune your daily habits. At the root of Ayurveda is its focus on the uniqueness of each individual. As such, it is a universal system applicable to anyone living in any part of the world. It is personalised medicine at its best.

Ayurveda is a wonderfully simple system to follow because it just requires you to be aware of the world around you. It's really a lesson in 'life-watching

and feeling'. Take the extremes in nature: is it hot or cold, wet or dry, light or heavy? How do these extremes affect and influence us? For example, the sun is hot and can give you life-sustaining Vitamin D or life-paining sunburn. Eczema is a 'hot' disease needing cooling anti-inflammatories while low thyroid is a 'cold' disease requiring stimulating hormonal balance. Some foods are hot, like whiskey and chillies, too much of which will probably lead to heartburn. As we start to notice and understand what is going on, we can begin to make a choice.

Ayurveda helps us make those choices by teaching us how to live according to our unique and individual constitutional make-up. You may well have heard about the three Ayurvedic constitutions: *vata*, *pitta* and *kapha*. These are called the three *dosha*. When our behaviour and environment support our *dosha*-tendencies we are healthy, when they don't, we can struggle.

Our *dosha* is really the Ayurvedic description of our genetic potential. We inherit from our ancestors the qualities and tendencies that make us unique. And by understanding these tendencies and their potential as well as limitations, we can influence the behaviour and performance of our cells. Ayurveda has grouped these tendencies into three general groups.

Vata (V)

Vata is connected with the elements of mobile wind and spacious space. It regulates movement and communication and relates to the nervous system. It's responsible for how anything and everything moves in and out of your body: breath, nutrition, nerves, hormones, flatus and foetus. *Vata* types are not the best at managing their resources, but they are the pinnacle of creative energy. Sensitive, aware and conscientious, they can overthink life and turn into a worry ball of anxiety.

If *vata* is out of balance then you may experience fluctuating energy, bouts of depression, insomnia, indigestion, constipation, painful periods, scanty periods or infertility. *Vata*'s health can be vulnerable to fluctuation, and while they can go down quickly they soon bounce back. Musicians, poets and mystics tend to be *vata*.

Pitta (P)

Pitta is connected with the elements of transformational fire and fluid water. It regulates heat, manages digestion and influences metabolic hormone production. *Pitta* is expert at managing energy, hence many of them are managers, athletes and people who get things done. However all this precision and perfection can lead to a bit of a hot collar and the occasional blown gasket when things don't go right. Naturally competitive with themselves, *pitta* types like to be better than everyone else. If out of balance, the result could be heartburn, high blood pressure, skin rashes, hot flushes and irritation. Blessed with robust health, they need to keep levels

of heat and inflammation down so they can channel their inherent compassionate nature and avoid blowing up.

Kapha (K)

Kapha is connected with the elements of solid earth and cohesive water. It is responsible for strength, moisture levels and the structure of the body. *Kapha*'s job is to store energy. They are the masters of conservation, which gives them huge brain power, great memories and remarkable stamina. Unfortunately, they often have a dislike for giving energy away, don't like change, avoid exercise and love the sofa a bit too much. If *kapha* is out of balance then holding too much weight, mucousy chest infections, sluggish energy and – in the longrun – congestive heart problems and diabetes aren't too far behind. As strong as *kapha* people get, they need to stay on the move to keep digestion and metabolism moving.

Ayurveda in health and disease

Just because some of us have largely discarded our traditional healing knowledge in favour of 'magic-bullet' medicine, this doesn't mean it's of no value and not thriving in other parts of the world. The traditional use of plants for healing is the refined knowledge of hundreds of generations. In true scientific investigatory style, it's been carefully evaluated and re-evaluated by the practitioners of that tradition again and again. It is not just the anecdotal accounts of a few practitioners or enthusiastic newbies. When traditional use is part of a great system and culture, the information it shares should be rated highly because it has evolved over many years and been tried on large numbers of people. As Ayurveda has grown up within Indian culture (which by all accounts can only be described as a great culture), its insights should also be highly rated as both reliable and useful. So should Chinese, Japanese and other traditions of natural healing.

Ayurveda teaches that disease is primarily due to an imbalance in the inner processes of the body and mind. In other words, the way in which we are responding to the challenges we face isn't supporting our health as best it could. This is different from our modern functional view of disease: that organs are in isolation from each other and microbes or hormones cause disease. It's that old 'terrain' versus 'germ' theory (that if the terrain is strong germs can't harm us). Although Ayurveda understands the potential of invading organisms that can overwhelm even the strongest constitution, its primary understanding of disease is systemic rather than reductionist. Disease, especially chronic disease, arises when a whole system is out of balance. Ayurveda focuses on patterns in physiology rather than just pathology. Ayurveda focuses on you and not just a number or the name of the disease.

If you want to learn more, then see my book inspired by Ayurveda, *A Pukka Life: Your Path to Perfect Health*, which goes into much more detail. But so you can understand a bit more about blending the right tea for you, here are how different tastes can influence our health.

The taste of nature

Nature is overflowing with a medley of flavours, and we are born ready to explore them all. We have 2,000 to 5,000 taste buds on our tongues with 100 receptors per bud. That's a lot of taste sensation centres. The different flavours are perceived through different molecular exchanges at the taste bud receptors. As well as our taste buds, other factors are also at work when it comes to our total experience of taste: our sense of smell enhances our taste experience, while nerves convey the experience of texture and temperature to our brains. The company helps too.

While modern science identifies just five tastes (sweet, sour, salty, bitter, umami), Ayurveda has long recognised six tastes. Along with sweet, salty, sour and bitter, it considers 'spicy-pungent' and 'astringent' as flavours. Spicy-pungency is experienced via nerve signals sent from the mouth (while chewing) to the brain, and astringency is experienced as a tightening of mucous membranes on the tongue and in the mouth caused by tannins in the food – because of this, they don't classify as 'official' tastes. But as Ayurveda is really a practical system (and by far the most developed system in the world for categorising the effects of taste on our health), it includes ones that have specific physiological effects.

The Sanskrit word for taste is *rasa*, and it is a very pregnant word: as well as 'taste', it can mean 'essence', 'juice', 'sap', 'lymphatic fluid', 'flavour' and 'delicious'. Just saying the word sounds 'juicy'. Flavour is the essence of life – it affects everything. And while I am on the subject of deliciousness, 'pukka' is a word that means 'genuine' and 'authentic', as well as also translating to 'juicy, ripe and ready to eat'.

To understand how taste works within Ayurveda, you need to learn some basic principles. These next few paragraphs are a bit more technical. Use this section as a reference as and when you need clarification.

Ayurveda teaches that everything on earth has all of the five natural elements – space, air, fire, water and earth – within it, but that usually only one or two are dominant. For example, the spicy-pungent flavour is energetically dominated by fire and air and, like a fire and the wind, the flavour is hot, drying and light. In addition to possessing elemental qualities, taste has a number of effects on the body and mind.

Temperature

Each specific taste affects the thermo-regulatory and metabolic qualities in the body (i.e. heating it up or cooling it down). For example, cinnamon is spicy-pungent and hot, which raises body temperature. Grapes are sweet and cooling, which can help cool you down.

Hot

Heat warms, dries, invigorates and stimulates the tissues. Just as the sun on a hot day causes the blood to come to the surface of the body, so energetically hot herbs cause our metabolism to expand upwards and outwards, opening the pores of the skin. Hot substances are high in the fire element. Heat increases the metabolism, encourages circulation, causes sweating, light-headedness and thirst. Hot substances are usually used to treat cold, contracted, hypo- and sluggish conditions. Beneficial to *kapha* and *vata*, it dries damp, phlegm and warms cold. As like increases like, spicy-pungent qualities in herbs like ginger or cinnamon strengthen the digestive fire (called *agni* in Ayurveda) to function at optimum level. Herbs that are heating usually contain volatile oils or mustard glycosides that stimulate gastric secretions as well as help the body assimilate nutrients. Hot-natured herbs and foods have a particular affinity with the heart, head, liver and lungs and are commonly used when these areas are imbalanced, but the hot substances may damage them if used injudiciously. Pungent, sour and salty herbs tend to be heating.

Cold

Cold-natured herbs cool, moisten and sedate the tissues and metabolism. Rather like the cold of a winter's day causes you to shiver energetically, cold herbs contract the muscles and narrow the channels of circulation. They are high in the water element. Cold substances are usually used to treat 'hot', inflamed and hyper- conditions. Cold benefits *pitta* while aggravating *kapha* and *vata*. Herbs that are cold-natured soothe painful and inflammatory heat conditions. Digestion is easily damaged by cold-natured herbs and should be used cautiously when there is diarrhoea and sluggish digestion from the cold. Cold herbs have an affinity with the stomach, the kidneys and the bladder and can weaken them if used excessively. Bitter, astringent and sweet herbs tend to be cooling.

Quality (heavy/light, wet/dry, penetrating/soft)

Taste also defines the effects of a particular herb or food. Whether it is light or heavy to digest, and wet or dry on the mucous membranes. It also defines whether the herb is penetrating or soft. For example, black pepper is spicy and hot as well as having the other qualities of being light, dry and penetrating: it is easy to digest, dries the mucous membranes and penetrates deeply into the tissues. Chew on a peppercorn and these qualities will become clear. Marshmallow root is the opposite: it is sweet and also moistening and soft, making it especially valuable for healing wounds and reducing dryness and inflammation. Try some and see.

Direction (where the food goes in the body)

Tastes also have an affinity with certain parts of the body. We all know that garlic goes to our lungs as we can smell it on our (and other people's) breath.

It's good for lung infections and coughs. Asparagus is renowned for making us pee – Ayurveda knows asparagus is a bitter and cooling food that clears internal heat via the urinary system. It's good for cystitis and urinary problems. Ginger has multiple 'sites', clearing mucus from the lungs, warming the skin, invigorating the blood and relaxing the muscles. Some herbs go to the brain (sage), some to the heart (hawthorn berry), some to the urinary system (corn silk), some to the skin (burdock root)... Knowing where a herb goes is one of the essential keys to really understanding how to blend herbs.

Additionally, taste has an effect on the movement of energy in the body, by influencing the direction that *vata* (the *dosha* responsible for movement) travels in. For example, the pungent taste (e.g. in fresh ginger) ascends and spreads energy outwards, causing sweating, while the bitter taste (e.g. in coffee) descends, causing energy to move downwards, with a diuretic and laxative effect.

Dosha (effect on the constitution)

Tastes also influence your *dosha*. For example, the sweet flavour builds earthy *kapha*, cools hot-*pitta* and reduces airy *vata*. As sweet is a nourishing taste, it increases the volume of all the tissues. Hence, it is no surprise that we live off sweet-tasting foods, like wheat, rice and vegetables, as they keep us strong.

We will now explore in depth the six tastes: sweet, sour, salty, spicy-pungent, bitter and astringent. As we do, it's worth keeping in mind that how we 'taste' life affects our health and mood. If your experience of life is 'sweet' you are usually happy, while 'bitter' episodes are less savoury. Because our taste of life becomes our *rasa*, our essence, it is helpful to learn how taste affects us so that we can keep it 'sweet'.

The Six Tastes

Sweet
The sweet flavour is made from the elements of earth and water. This means that it has the qualities of these two building blocks: heavy and descending (like earth) and, like water, it is wet and cold (when water is subjected to heat it becomes hot, but in its 'primordial' state it is cold). A bit like making sand-castles, when we mix earth and water it creates a sticky goo that can hold everything together. Sweet is the taste of strength and structure. It is also the flavour of love, of sharing and of compassion. We give sweets to friends as an act of sharing and companionship. It is considered the most spiritually nourishing of flavours and is used to heighten experience of clarity and awareness of the spiritual aspect of life.

We all know the sweet flavour. Its main receptors are at the front of the tongue. Sweet comes from sugars: glucose, sucrose, fructose, maltose. They are made up of short (mono) and long (poly) chains of saccharides. It is the flavour of energy. Many carbohydrates, fats and proteins are sweet and their potential energy is measured in kilajoules. Foods and herbs with the sweet flavour are considered to be tonics, and they build and nourish all the tissues. Licorice (*Glycyrrhiza glabra*), beetroot (*Beta vulgaris*) and shatavari (*Asparagus racemosus*) are sweet and nourish the deeper reproductive tissues. The sweet flavour increases reproductive strength and the integrity of the immune system. Many renowned immune tonics have a sweet flavour and are full of immune-modulating saponins and polysaccharides.

Sweet substances and experiences increase fluid-*kapha* and reduce hot-*pitta* and nervous-*vata*. As a *demulcent*, soft, soothing and wet flavour, sweet reduces some of the dryness and weakness associated with *vata*. It is a tissue healer, and sweet herbs are often used for hastening wound repair (such as aloe vera or marshmallow). Sweet benefits the mucous membranes lining the mouth, lungs, digestive, urinary and reproductive systems. The sweet taste can help to clear a dry throat and lungs by enhancing *expectoration*. Its cooling anti-inflammatory tendencies help to remove the intense heat of *pitta* or '-itis' conditions (like bronchitis). This is also helped by its softening, mild laxative effect. It benefits the complexion, improves hair and nail quality and is the best flavour for a smooth voice. Following the principle of like increases like, you want to increase your sweet experiences and flavours in life in order to be truly nourished, loved and cherished. This will create a cycle of ever-increasing benevolence.

Used in concentrated excess, such as with refined sugar/pastries/ice creams, it can increase mucus and promote congestion. It can cause toxins (called *ama* in Ayurveda), fever, chest and breathing problems, swollen lymph glands, flaccidity, heaviness, worms, fungal infections, obesity and diabetes. Exceptions to this rule of sweet substances increasing *kapha* are honey, mung beans and barley; they are actually considered to balance excess moisture as they can be diuretic.

Because sweet is the taste of life, many of our Pukka teas and remedies are sweet: Three Licorice, Three Fennel, Three Cinnamon, Peppermint and Licorice, Licorice and Cinnamon, Vanilla Chai, Elderberry and Echinacea, Chamomile, Vanilla and Manuka Honey, Detox, Relax, Refresh, Night Time, Blackcurrant Beauty, Sweet Vanilla Green and Love, as well as the Elderberry Syrup, Vitalise, Clean Greens and Aloe Vera Juice.

Sour

The sour flavour is made from the elements of earth and fire. Its qualities are hot, oily and light. It creates both dampness and heat in the body and mind. It stimulates digestion and clears dryness. Sour foods make the mouth moist and increase the flow of saliva. When taken in excess sour draws the tissues inwards and 'puckers' the lips and makes your hairs stand on end. This contraction creates an emotional reluctance to share things. Eating too much sour flavoured food is believed to encourage envy and can make your experience of life feel sour.

The sour flavour is found in acids: citric, lactic, malic, oxalic and ascorbic. The receptors for the sour- flavour are found on taste buds on the sides of the tongue. The acids have a direct effect on digestion by promoting liver function through various mechanisms. As sour flavours can reduce stomach acid it also means that the liver needs to produce less acid- neutralising alkaline fluids. Sour flavours also increase the flow of bile that helps to encourage digestion of fats. Unripe fruits are sour and are commonly used as digestive chutneys in India. Sour fruits such as lemons and amalaki are high in Vitamin C and are considered to be antioxidant, rejuvenating and tonic herbs.

As the sour flavour aggravates hot-*pitta* and liquefies sticky-*kapha* it is not usually beneficial in hot and damp conditions. It is also considered to irritate the blood, and people with skin diseases are recommended to avoid it. Most fermented foods are sour – fermented yoghurt, sourdough breads, vinegar, pickles and alcohol are sour foods that increase heat and mucus in the body. Anyone who has drunk one too many glasses of wine can tell you that. Sour nourishes all the tissues bar the deepest reproductive tissue. It alleviates *vata* and aggravations of the of the nervous system, and it draws scattered energy back in. It is a specific *carminative* useful for promoting digestion, while also removing gas and indigestion. Amalaki, lemons and pomegranate seeds are the exception to the rule that the sour flavour aggravates *pitta*, as they actually reduce heat and inflammation.

In excess, sour can cause dizziness, thirst, burning sensations, fever, itching, anaemia and skin diseases.

The Pukka teas and remedies with a few sour flavour notes are Lemon and Mandarin, Clean Greens, Detox with Lemon, Blackcurrant Beauty, Elderberry and Echinacea, Womankind, as well as Natural Vitamin C, Wholistic Triphala and Womankind Cranberry supplements.

Salty

Salt is predominantly made from the water and fire elements. It creates moisture and heat and is heavy and sinking. A grain dropped onto the tongue is instantly moistening. A sprinkle on food kindles digestion. It is an easily recognisable flavour and its receptors are towards the front of the tongue. Its sinking and heavy effect is very grounding for the nervous system, and this encourages stability. People who are solid and reliable become known as 'the salt of the earth'.

The use of salt is a good lesson in the importance of dosage. In correct quantities it is vital to our very existence and is as essential to our health as water and food. It can save lives when there is dehydration. In contrast to this, a sprinkle too much will cause an ulcer and aggravate stomach acidity. Excess salt consumption also causes water retention, with the accompanying results of puffy skin, oedema and even high blood pressure. This physical 'holding' is reflected in salt's emotional effects, as it causes greediness and encourages the desire for more flavour. To repeat the famous Ayurvedic adage, it is all about who is taking how much, of what and when.

Salt is found in minerals, and there are eight types of salt mentioned in Ayurveda, including rock, sea, black and pink. Rock is considered the best as it is very high in minerals and, unlike the other salts, does not cause as much water retention and it is not detrimental to the eyes.

Salty is the rarest flavour in the Ayurvedic repertoire of herbs, and is not found in many herbs. It is found in shilajit, a natural mineral rock exudate, full of numerous nourishing minerals. Seaweeds and celery are other examples of the salty flavour.

Salt aggravates hot-*pitta* and wet-*kapha*. It also disrupts the blood and is not recommended for people with skin diseases or bleeding problems. Its use in marinades reflects its softening quality, and it is used to soften masses, as well as a *demulcent* to liquefy *kapha*. It alleviates any excess of tired and dry *vata* by stimulating the appetite, moistening dryness and nourishing the nervous system. It is a mild laxative at a medium dose (3g) and an emetic that makes you throw up at higher dose (5–10g).

In excess it causes ulcers, skin diseases, grey hair, baldness and thirst.

Pukka's saltiest teas and remedies are high in minerals such as Cleanse, Supreme Matcha Green, as well as our super-herb blends of Vitalise, Clean Greens, Juicy Wheat Grass, Spirulina and Chlorella.

Pungent

The pungent flavour is a combination of the fire and air elements. Its qualities are hot, dry and light as well as penetrating and ascending. The acrid heat of hot foods and spices spreads throughout the whole system. Too much heat, whether climatic

About Ayurveda

from passion and excitement to anger and irritation. It is the most volatile of the tastes.

It is primarily found in the aromatic volatile oils, resins, oleo-resins and mustard glycosides. All these compounds are used to stimulate, invigorate, dry and clear the accumulation of wet, stagnant and congestive conditions. The essential oils of ginger and black pepper are often used for clearing mucus congestion or warming a cold condition. Pungent resins such as guggul and frankincense also invigorate the flow of blood, scrape out toxins and reduce cholesterol. The aromatic cardamom is an excellent digestive for encouraging sluggish digestion. Unlike the other tastes it does not have a specific taste bud receptor site but works through irritation of local tissue and nerve endings.

Pungent herbs and foods are a panacea for *kapha* as they dry the excess moisture and mucus so prevalent in this humour. Pungent herbs are vital for any weight-loss programme as they stimulate the metabolism and reduce fat. They directly cook and burn toxic-*ama* (unmetabolised wastes) as well as also clearing it via sweating. The heat encourages dilatation of the pores of the skin, causing the body to sweat, therefore throwing off unmetabolised toxins through the skin. When used in high volumes, the pungent flavour usually increases *vata* but, in moderation, it can also help to remove the cold stiffness of *vata* while encouraging healthy digestion. The heat of pungent herbs irritates *pitta* and should not usually be used where there is inflammation, especially with aggravation of the plasma (*rasa*) and blood (*rakta*) tissues. Its drying effect on bodily fluids can cause constipation.

In excess it creates burning, dizziness, thirst and excessive dryness. Ginger and cooked garlic are the exceptions to the rule that pungent flavours aggravate *vata*. In fact, they benefit it as they increase digestion and reduce intestinal gases.

Pukka's spiciest teas are Three Ginger, Three Cinnamon, Original Chai, Revitalise, Licorice and Cinnamon, Lemongrass and Ginger, Wild Apple and Cinnamon, Three Tulsi, and Three Mint, as well as After Dinner, Natural Balance and ManPlus supplements.

Bitter
This therapeutically priceless taste is created from a combination of space and air elements. Its dominant qualities are cooling, drying and light. It creates space in the body by draining and drying excess fluids. Too many bitter herbs can literally 'space you out' and leave you feeling disorientated. Many psychotropics are bitter, such as the 'magic' gilled mushroom genus Psilocybe. It has a particular affinity with the blood.

Bitters are usually classified as *alteratives* as they alter the chemical balance of the blood by clearing toxins. As they encourage the flow of bile and the activity of the liver this may account for some of bitter's detoxifying activity. Too much bitter flavour can weaken the kidneys, cause excess urination and emotionally encourages fear and anxiety. The bitter flavour has a negative effect on the strength of *kapha* and *ojas* (vigour) which reside in the heart. Again, it is all about an accurate diagnosis and using an appropriate dose for each individual person.

In Western herbalism bitters are associated with a tonic effect, in Ayurveda they are considered depleting. The tonic association comes from the low-dose, digestive-stimulating and liver-promoting perspective. The depleting and cleansing view comes from the experience that relatively larger doses of bitter herbs are cooling, reducing, detoxifying, laxative and diuretic. Studying and applying the insights of herbalism is a constant reminder to be specific. Everything is unique: how you apply the medicine, when you apply it, to whom it is applied and where it is administered all have an effect. Ayurveda clearly teaches that any substance can be a food, a medicine or a poison depending on how much is given, who is eating it, when it is eaten and where it is taken.

The reason that the bitter flavour is found in plants is often attributed to its ability to defend itself. If you taste nasty, no one will eat you! The bitter taste receptors are at the back of the tongue, and are the body's way of giving us a last line of defence. The bitter flavour is found in sesquiterpenes, anthraquinones, alkaloids and some glycosides. Plants with these properties are renowned for their anti-inflammatory, antimicrobial, anti-pyretic and digestive secretion-enhancing activities. These compounds are usually found intermixed with pungent and aromatic or astringent-tasting plants. Our humble dandelion has a very bitter leaf and a mildly bitter root, while neem, andrographis and chamomile are well-known bitters famed for their ability to clear infection, heal skin problems and purify the blood.

Bitter herbs clear sticky-*kapha* and inflammed-*pitta* while aggravating dry-*vata*. Excess dampness and heat are reduced as the bitter flavour drains them out of the system. Bitters also promote peristaltic rhythmical movements (contraction and relaxation) in the bowels as well as promoting urination. They are often indicated in lung conditions, especially with infections manifesting with green and sticky mucus. They excel at clearing itching, swelling and oozing on the skin.

A little is used as a stimulant to the appetite as the light quality can enhance the digestion and clear the palate. Higher doses are used to kill worms and parasites in the intestines and blood. Bitter herbs also benefit people who are overweight as they can dry and scrape away the adhesions and fatty accumulations.

When misused or incorrectly prescribed they can cause too much dryness and wasting in the body and mind – this can upset the nervous system, causing constipation, dizziness, weakness, reduction in semen and dryness of the whole body. Guduchi is a bitter herb that is an exception to the above as, along with the bitter benefits, it is also an aphrodisiac.

Pukka's teas and supplements with some bitter notes are Supreme Matcha Green, Three Chamomile, After Dinner, Detox, and also Andrographis, Wholistic Neem, Glow and Illuminate supplements.

Astringent
Astringent is the driest flavour. Made from a predominance of the earth and air elements, it is heavy, cold and dry. On eating something astringent your whole mouth contracts and draws the mucous membranes closer together. Astringency holds things in place and is used for prolapse, weakening muscles and loss of skin tone. However, having too much can leave you with a lack of taste for life and even resentful at its lack of zest.

The astringent flavour is found in tannins. These polyphenols are particularly concentrated in the bark, leaves and outer rind of fruits of plants and trees. They appear to offer some form of outer protection by repairing wounds and neutralising bacteria. They are especially soluble in water – think of the drying nature of a strong cup of tea left to steep for too long. Astringency is often found in combination with plants that also taste sweet or sour. Tea, haritaki and raspberry leaf are notably astringent.

Therapeutically the astringent flavour clears mucus-*kapha* and irritated-*pitta* while its dryness aggravates an already dry *vata*. It is very useful where there is any leakage of body fluids: bleeding (externally and internally), excessive sweating, involuntary urination, diarrhoea, excess catarrh, discharge in women and premature ejaculation. It holds tissues together, and astringent herbs are often used as a wash to help heal wounds. This holding effect also prevents loose and flaccid tissue from accumulating. Using astringent herbs is appropriate to treat sinking problems such as prolapses. Its effect on the digestive system benefits diarrhoea by astringing the bowel and stopping excessive downward flow. This also helps absorption by drawing fluids and nutrients inwards. Astringents are used for *pitta* inflammations to draw the swelling inwards, cool the heat and also drying any damp pus forming.

These dry, rough and light qualities are similar to *vata*. Because astringent tastes contract the tissues and obstruct the flow of *prana* (also known as the life-force) and nervous energy in the system it is detrimental to *vata*. In excess it can cause *vata* diseases like rigidity, pain in the heart, convulsions and retention of gas, urine and faeces.

Pukka's teas and remedies with the most astringency are Elegant English Breakfast, Gorgeous Earl Grey, Original Chai, Supreme Matcha Green, Rooibos and Honeybush, Three Cinnamon, as well as Wholistic Triphala, Triphala Plus and Natural Balance supplements.

Tastes and qualities			
Taste	Element	Quality	Effect on *dosha*
Sweet	Earth, Water	Heavy, Wet, Cold	K+ P– V–
Sour	Earth, Fire	Heavy, Wet, Warm	K+ P+ V–
Salty	Water, Fire	Heavy, Wet, Warm	K+ P+ V+
Pungent	Fire, Air	Light, Dry, Warm	K– P+ V+
Bitter	Space, Air	Light, Dry, Cold	K– P– V+
Astringent	Air, Earth	Light, Dry, Cold	K– P– V+

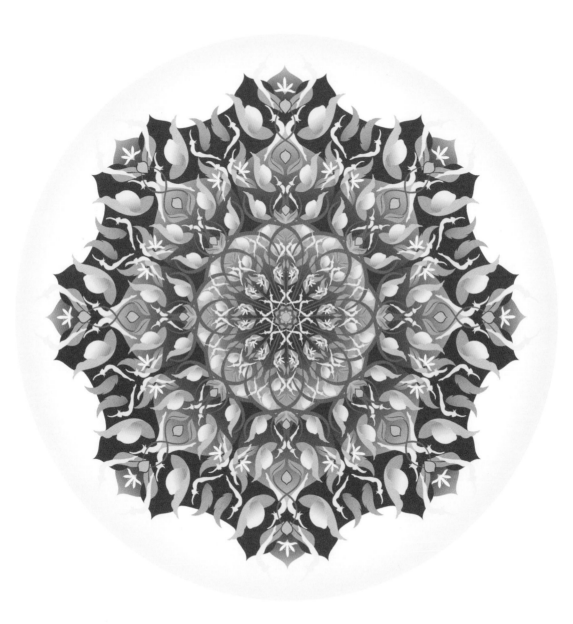

About Ayurveda

Pukkapedia

Aloe vera *Aloe barbadensis* The inner leaf gel of aloe vera is cooling and soothing with powerful anti-inflammatory properties. It has an affinity with the blood and skin, reducing any redness and heat. It influences the digestive system and the female reproductive system where it cools inflamed mucosal membranes (around organs) and regulates the blood flow.

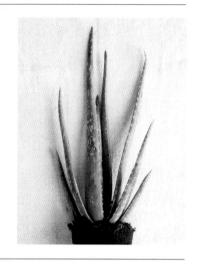

Almond *Prunus dulcis* Sweet to taste, heating, heavy and oily in quality, this nut is a building, strengthening and aphrodisiac tonic that boosts fertility. Almonds are the most superior nut, also benefiting the lungs, skin and digestive tract. Soak overnight to remove their *pitta*-irritating skin and turn them into an enzyme-rich superfood.

Amla fruit *Phyllanthus emblica* Restorative to the immune system, amla provides support and nourishment to the body after prolonged infections. It also has an affinity with the blood and will help to cleanse the system from circulating heat-toxins (spots, skin rashes) and contains antioxidant properties.

Angelica, Chinese *Angelica sinensis* A potent, nutrient-rich tonic that helps to replenish and build blood. It is quite aromatic, and its warming nature quickens the flow of blood, bringing colour to the cheeks. Do not use in pregnancy without the guidance of a herbalist.

Aniseed *Pimpinella anisum* A *carminative* for the digestive system and an effective antispasmodic for colic pain, bloating and indigestion.

Ashwagandha root *Withania somnifera* A deeply nourishing *vata*-balancing herb that gently rebuilds strength. It is helpful for assisting deep sleep and calming nervous *vata*. Its ability to replenish the blood, enhance nutrients and build bone strength make it indispensable in disorders of degeneration and ageing. Its affinity with the adrenal, endocrine and nervous systems points to its use in any imbalances affecting energy or vitality. I think Ashwagandha is the perfect herb for the 21st century as it calms and energises. It builds while also helping us adapt to the stresses of life. Do not use in pregnancy without the guidance of a herbalist.

Astragalus root *Astragalus membranaceus* One of traditional Chinese herbalism's great tonics. It raises the *qi*, replenishing the life-force. It is specific for raising white blood cells to help the immune system fight infections. People with a more delicate nature might use it to make them more robust.

Beetroot *Beta vulgaris* Packed with iron, calcium and Vitamin A and C, beetroot is very nutritious. It also contains a pigment known as betanin, which is a strong detoxifier for the liver and is a blood builder.

Bhringraj leaf *Eclipta alba* A restorative to the tissues, but particularly the scalp and hair follicles, this leaf encourages hair growth. Bhringraj improves the blood supply to the brain and clears sinus congestion. It treats mental anxiety and tension that can be linked with chronic insomnia and also encourages the production of bile and improved metabolic processes within the liver.

Bibhitaki *Terminalia bellirica* This is an astringent and *expectorant*, which strengthens the mucous membranes in

Black pepper seed *Piper nigrum*
This enhances nutrient absorption and digestive enzyme activity. It stimulates the capillaries, thereby enhancing detoxification and nutrient transportation.

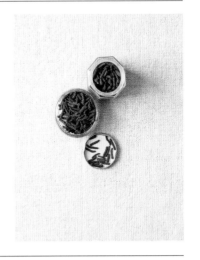

the body. It effectively clears congestion in the lungs and digestive tract.

Bilberry *Vaccinium myrtillus* Bilberries are full of antioxidants, which help to scavenge free radicals. It is very effective for eye health, improving the blood supply to them while strengthening the walls of the capillaries.

Boswellia resin A natural painkiller specific for inflammation and swelling. It contains boswellic acid – an active component that reduces pain and inflammation. It stimulates circulation and removes stagnation and congestion such as cholesterol. Do not use in pregnancy without the guidance of a herbalist.

Buchu leaf *Agathosma betulina* A South African herb that is powerfully antimicrobial in the urinary tract. It is a diuretic and can help clear infections.

Burdock root *Arctium lappa* Burdock is a bitter and cleansing *alterative*. It reduces inflammation and improves the circulation of fluids around the body, nourishing and cleansing the tissues. It also contains antimicrobial components (polyacetylenes), which are particularly effective for helping skin infections. Burdock improves oil secretion in the skin, which cleanses and clears the sebaceous glands.

Cardamom *Elletaria cardamomum* Highly aromatic, cardamom is an effective *carminative* to the digestive system, providing relief from the symptoms of indigestion. It stimulates metabolic and digestive processes while also working as a decongestant, removing mucus from the digestive and respiratory tracts.

Catnip leaf *Nepeta cataria* A calming *diaphoretic* used for breaking a fever and easing digestion. Often found in children's immunity teas because it is gently effective.

Celery seed *Apium graveolens* A stimulating and cooling diuretic, celery seed penetrates and breaks down accumulated uric acid deposits and then eliminates them from the body through the improvement of blood flow to and through the kidneys. Celery's ability to improve blood flow also means that it cleanses the joints and cartilage by increasing the level of fluid moving through them.

Chamomile flower *Matricaria recutita* These exquisite and useful yellow flowers are full of sweetness that can help to relax the nervous system. Chamomile is often used as a tasty tea to induce good sleep, settle restless legs and stop spasms. It also has a mild bitter flavour that makes it a wonderful digestive, easing bloating, cramps and inflammation throughout the digestive system. Chamomile is not to be confused with Roman Chamomile (*Anthemis nobilis*), which is much more bitter in flavour.

Corn silk *Zea mays* This strengthens the muscle tone in the urethra. It is a *demulcent* which promotes the healing and soothing of the protective mucosa membrane that lines the urinary tract. It is sweet, soothing and soft.

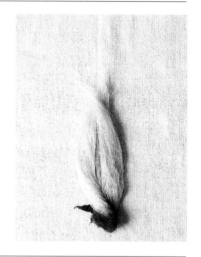

Chicory root *Cichorium intybus*
Chicory's bitter compounds benefit the liver – roasted chicory becomes even more effective and has a rich nutty taste.

Chlorella *Chlorella pyrenoidosa*
A supreme detoxifier, chorella naturally cleanses the whole body. It is able to cleanse heavy metals as well as help alkalise. It also contains Chlorella Growth Factor, a remarkable component that encourages normal cell growth and renewal.

Chrysanthemum flower
Chrysanthemum morifolium
Bright, light and loving the eyes, chrysanthemum's mild bitterness helps clear heat from the head. It's useful for mild headaches and inflamed eyes.

Cinnamon bark *Cinnamomum aromaticum* This protects and strengthens the intestines, balances blood sugar levels and also has an

antifungal compound that acts upon yeast and fungal infections in addition to balancing the gut flora. Cinnamon's warm and spicy nature also gently stimulates circulation.

Cocoa bean *Theobroma cacao*
High in theobromine which relaxes the nervous system. It is also very high in flavonoids, which are potent antioxidants that protect against free radicals.

Coriander seed *Coriandrum sativum*
This kindles the digestive fire, improving the efficiency of metabolic and digestive processes. Coriander also has antibacterial and antispasmodic properties.

Cramp bark *Viburnum opulus* A potent antispasmodic, cramp bark helps ease menstrual pain and stops involuntary muscular spasm. It has a particular affinity with the uterus and is also useful for spasmodic coughs, headaches and general muscular spasms and pain.

Cranberry *Vaccinium oxycoccus*
A urinary antiseptic that prevents the adhesion of bacteria to the bladder, therefore protecting against repeated infections. Cranberry also breaks down calcium carbonate and calculi in the urinary system and the kidneys.

Cumin seed *Cuminum cyminum*
A *carminative* to the digestive system, improving metabolic processes and the ability to absorb nutrients more effectively. Cumin also has strong antispasmodic qualities – helpful where there may be colic or indigestion.

Damiana leaf *Turnera diffusa* As a relaxing *nervine*, damiana can help 'stage fright' caused by impending intimacy. It's a gentle antidepressant that lifts your mood and helps you feel more like you.

Dandelion root and leaf *Taraxacum officinale* A superb diuretic that cleanses the body without depleting it. It is considered to be one of the finest

Elderberry & elderflower *Sambucus nigra*

A strong antiviral and antibacterial that effectively treats colds and flu. It deactivates the virus and strengthens the cell membranes so that we are better able to resist a virus's proliferation. Elderberry has a particular affinity for treating respiratory conditions, removing congestion and mucus from the respiratory tract. The flower is more diffusive, helping to bring on a sweat when there is fever or reduce hayfever when there is an allergy.

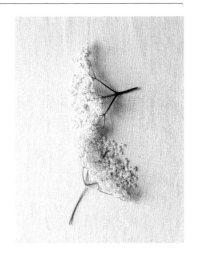

remedies for the liver and blood, reducing toxicity and stagnation. Dandelion has a particular strength for removing deep-seated heat and inflammation that has become embedded in the system. The leaf is renowned for aiding the urinary system while the root has more affinity with the liver and skin.

Echinacea root and leaf *Echinacea purpurea* Traditionally used as an antidote to poisonous snake bites, echinacea is a powerful immune stimulant. It supports the body's ability to ward off bacterial and viral infections, cleanses the lymphatic system and is a powerful anti-inflammatory. It contains alkamides that create a typical echinacea tongue tingle.

Fennel seed *Foeniculum vulgare* This contains anethole, which has strong anti-inflammatory properties. Fennel is a superb *carminative* to the digestive system and is also a strong antimicrobial and antifungal agent.

Flower pollen A renowned energy nutrient high in essential proteins and amino acids. This wonderful golden grain has all the known nutrients necessary for human survival. It is gathered by bees from the stamens of flowers and collected from hives as small pellets. It contains approximately 35 per cent vegetable protein, around 18 vitamins, 25 minerals, 60 trace elements and all amino acids. It is also full of enzymes, co-enzymes, growth hormones, essential fatty acids and slow-releasing carbohydrates. Pollen is extremely rich in Vitamins B (including B12), C, D and E, and in lecithin, cysteine and golden yellow carotenes, which are metabolic precursors of Vitamin A.

Galangal root *Alpinia galanga* This member of the ginger family is rich in volatile oils that give it a very special lemony-gingery-spicy and hot flavour. Traditionally used for throat, immune and digestive problems, it's also an effective painkiller for back pain and headaches.

Ghee Ghee contains a balance of easy-to-digest, short-chain fatty acids that are essential for healthy skin, nerves and cells. Specifically, it lubricates the tissues, clears toxins and is an all-round rejuvenator. It is ideal for healthy cooking due to its high smoke point, which means it does not produce damaging free radicals and, when eaten as part of a vegetarian diet, it can help raise healthy HDL cholesterol and reduce bad LDL. Cooling and sweet, oily and heavy, clarified butter kindles the digestive fire (*agni*) and balances all three *dosha*s, but should not be used in *kapha* conditions with clear, white discharges and/or when there is general congestion.

Ginger root *Zingiber officinale* Warming and spicy with thermogenic properties that increase metabolism. It is anti-inflammatory and antioxidant making it pro-health. It contains constituents such as gingerols and shogaols, natural plant-protectors which have been shown to stimulate the circulation and reduce the stickiness of our blood platelets to give

Ginseng root *Panax ginseng* Red ginseng is primarily an *adaptogen* that nourishes the adrenal glands and acts upon the HPA (hypothalamic-pituitary-adrenal) axis. *Adaptogens* improve the body's ability to cope with stress by altering the release of stress hormones. Ginseng root enhances muscular strength and recovery by increasing the capacity of skeletal muscle to oxidise free fatty acids to produce cellular energy.

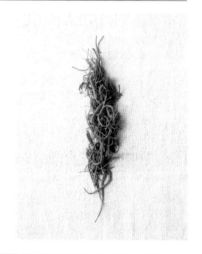

blood a healthier profile. Shogaols have anti-emetic properties, making ginger renowned for treating nausea.

Goji berry *Lycium chinensis* This red delight is a powerful rejuvenator for the eyes, skin and kidneys. Goji berry is a renowned blood tonic helping to bring nutrition to the organs and replenishing fluids where there is dryness (in all of the tissues in the body) and general weakness.

Gokshura fruit *Tribulus terrestris* A diuretic that also soothes the membranes of the urinary tract. It is a herb specific for the treatment of prostate conditions and it encourages the removal of obstructions in the kidneys and urinary system. In addition, it also strengthens and tonifies the reproductive system.

Gotu kola leaf *Centella asiatica*
This stimulates blood flow in the capillaries and reduces congestion in the veins while also strengthening the walls of the blood

vessels, making it an excellent wound healer for the skin. Gotu kola contains active compounds triterpene saponins known as asiaticosides that are considered important for circulating blood in the brain and enhancing trauma healing.

Green tea leaf *Camellia sinensis*
This is famed for its antioxidant properties, high polyphenol levels and green tea catechins including the famous EGCG (epigallocatechin gallate). These compounds give it the ability to combat free radicals and improve cellular health. Matcha, oolong, jasmine tea and black tea all come from the same green tea plant, *Camellia sinensis*.

Haritaki fruit *Terminalia chebula*
This contains sennosides, which are effective laxative agents. It also contains tannins, which are astringents and are effective against diarrhoea. It treats parasitic infections of the gut and helps encourage a healthy response to inflammation. Haritaki also reduces lipid

deposits in the blood, helping to reduce cholesterol levels.

Hawthorn berry *Crataegus monogyna*
Primarily a tonic for the heart, hawthorn improves the blood supply to the organ and increases the efficiency of the cardiac muscle, especially where there is damage and/or degeneration. Hawthorn will also help to regulate blood pressure.

Hemp seed oil *Cannabis sativa*
Sweet, cooling, heavy and unctuous, this balances all three *doshas*. The seed of this infamous plant is a superb *demulcent* laxative. It also has a perfect balance of omega-3, -6 and -9 essential fatty acids, and is high in Gamma Linolenic Acid (GLA) and Stearidonic Acid, making it an anti-inflammatory, nervous system restorative and cardiac tonic.

Holy basil *see* Tulsi leaf

Horsetail *Equesitum arvense* One of our most ancient plants, horsetail is a

Hops strobile *Humulus lupulus* A bitter and cooling relaxing sedative you can feel entering the nervous system. It helps you sleep and reduces anxiety. It has mild oestrogen regulating properties making it valuable for alleviating the symptoms of menopause.

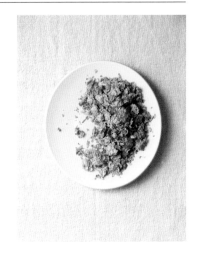

mineral accumulator packed with silica, valuable for strengthening skin, hair and nails. It's also useful for the urinary system.

Lavender flower *Lavandula angustifolia, spp.* Lavender moves stuck emotions by helping us feel present. As it creates a feeling of safety and trust, it lets us shed our worries and enjoy the moment. It is a favourite for helping to relieve insomnia, anxiety and the winter blues.

Lemon *Citrus x limon* Fresh lemon is naturally high in bioflavonoids and Vitamin C which protect the capillaries and strengthen the immune system. They are also effective at removing toxins from the blood and clearing congestion. The sour nature of lemons stimulates digestive processes and also the production of bile.

Lemon verbena *Aloysia citrodora* This delicate leaf has gentle anxiolytic (anti-anxiety) properties that help us stay calm and centred. Its natural opening effects help us to breathe deep and think clearly.

Lemongrass leaf *Cymbopogon citratus* This tough and fragrant grass exudes citrus aromas. It's very good for opening the chest, clearing mucus as well as removing a muzzy-headed feeling. Its also a potent *galactagogue*, helping the flow of breast milk.

Licorice root *Glycyrrhiza glabra* A sweet and soothing herb. It is primarily an *expectorant* and *demulcent*, removing congestion and mucus from the body, but also moistening and coating damaged and irritated mucous membranes. Licorice is a strong anti-inflammatory as well as a deep nourishing tonic.

Limeflower *Tilia argentea* Soft, sweet and delicate, limeflower is a wonderful relaxant to the whole nervous system, helping to reduce anxiety, bring a restful sleep as well as reduce blood pressure.

Linseed *Linum usitatissimum* A *demulcent* for the digestive system helping to soothe inflammation and

lubricate the bowels. Linseed produces prostaglandins that encourage a healthy response to inflammation.

Maca root *Lepidium meyenii* This improves mental acuity, physical endurance, vitality and stamina. It is known as an aphrodisiac tonic and used to increase libido as well as improve sperm and egg health.

Manuka honey Renowned for its antiviral and antibacterial qualities, manuka's unctuous nature soothes the throat and lungs, encouraging healing and repair.

Marigold petal *Calendula officinalis* Also known as calendula, this golden floret is one of nature's best wound healers for trauma caused internally and externally. It is a gentle *emmenagogue* (stimulates blood flow to the pelvic area), helping ease menstrual flow and prevent pain. Its wound healing properties go a long way toward healing gastric ulcers as well as lung inflammation.

Lemon balm *Melissa officinalis* It's all in the name... this 'balm' rapidly brings a sense of peace to a furrowed brow. It moves *prana* in your chest removing feelings of stagnation, especially for people who sigh a lot. It benefits digestion, menstrual cramps and calms the heart by regulating palpitations.

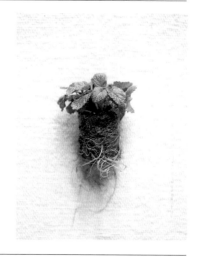

Motherwort leaf *Leonurus cardiaca*
A heart tonic that calms nervousness associated with female hormonal change and is particularly effective at treating palpitations. It contains aromatic and acrid bitters that calm the nervous system and relax the female reproductive system.

Neem leaf *Azadirachta indica* A strong blood purifier and anti-inflammatory. It is antibacterial and antifungal due to the constituent azadirachtin. It is effective in inflammatory conditions of the skin and digestive tract. Do not use in pregnancy without the guidance of a herbalist.

Nettle leaf *Urtica dioica* A nutritious plant filled with vitamins, minerals and protein. Nettle is excellent at ridding the body of excess proteinaceous waste, including those that build up in inflammatory conditions such as arthritis.

Nutmeg *Myristica fragrans* Known as a temporal sedative, nutmeg helps you stay asleep if you are prone to waking up in the middle of the night. Its *carminative* and hypotensive (lowering blood pressure) actions make it useful in formulas for aiding sleep. It is warming and astringent, which helps to hold your energy in your core.

Oat straw flowering top *Avena sativa*
Long used for restoring energy in cases of nervous exhaustion, oat straw is sweet, nourishing and replenishing for those suffering depression, frazzled nerves or headaches.

Passion flower *Passiflora incarnata*
This creeper climbs through our nervous system bringing peace, calm and clarity. It's a favourite for helping to ease insomnia caused by too much worry and mental stress. It is also a useful antispasmodic.

Pomegranate fruit *Punica granatum*
This has strong antioxidant properties. Pomegranate also tonifies and strengthens the cardiovascular system and reduces the build-up of cholesterol.

Psyllium husk *Plantago ovata*
A *demulcent* laxative soothing inflammatory digestive disorders and constipation.

Raspberry leaf *Rubus idaeus* A favoured herb of midwives, raspberry leaf is astringent and tones muscle. It is the most commonly used herb that is specific for harnessing uterine strength in preparation for labour. It is also used for stopping diarrhoea and bringing tone to the mucous membranes.

Red clover *Trifolium pratense*
An important phyto-oestrogenic plant containing isoflavones, which are classically used in the treatment of menopausal symptoms. Its oestrogen-regulating effects support women's health by improving bone density and cardiovascular health. It also reduces the risk of excessive oestrogen levels influencing irregular cellular growth.

Mint leaves *Mentha spp.* The aromatic leaf is famous for easing spasms and digestive discomfort. Mint is a good example of how helping your stomach can help your mind, as both areas in your body are responsible for digesting experiences. A cup of mint tea instantly strengthens digestion and clears your mind leaving you feeling revitalised and refreshed. Generally sweet, cooling and light, mints also balance all three *doshas*.

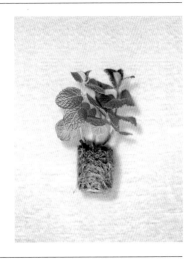

Rose flower *Rosa damascena*
A heart-opening favourite, rose is mildly astringent, helping to hold awareness in your centre (your heart). Use it to lift mild depression and open you to the possibility of love. Rose is also helpful for toning the tissues and organs and to stop bleeding, especially when associated with any emotional upset.

Rosehip *Rosa canina* Rosehip is a fantastic source of bioflavonoids and Vitamin C that help to boost the immune system. Rosehip also encourages a healthy response to inflammation.

Rosemary leaf *Rosmarinus officinalis*
Rosemary is a circulatory and nervous system stimulant but has a particular effect upon cerebral circulation, helping to improve cognitive processes such as memory and concentration. It also tones and calms the digestion, particularly where digestive processes are affected by anxiety.

Saffron *Crocus sativus* This is the most expensive spice, but potentially the most beneficial. Its colour points to its benefit for the blood. Saffron has a long tradition of treating heart problems, relieving menstrual pain and lifting your mood. Its high water-soluble carotenoid levels give it a potent antioxidant capacity. It is sweet, astringent, bitter, heating, dry and light – saffron reduces all three *doshas*.

Sage leaf *Salvia officinalis*
This is a much favoured herb for keeping the mind as sharp as the mind of a sage. It also stops leakage of fluids, so it is often used to stop sweating.

Schisandra berries *Schisandra chinensis* Also known as the five flavoured herb or *wu wei zi* in Chinese, schisandra is a liver-protecting herb that regulates the organ's detoxifying mechanisms.

Seaweed This has a diverse range of essential macro nutrients (such as proteins and carbohydrates) and micro nutrients (including iodine and calcium), and is one of the most nutritious forms of vegetation on the entire planet, facilitating and improving the absorption of other nutrients in our bodies.

Senna leaf *Senna alexandrina* A potent laxative that contains anthraquinones, which help to drain the bowel and clear intestinal heat. It should be used with caution and not more than a couple of weeks at a time.

Shatavari root *Asparagus racemosus*
A superb tonic for the female reproductive system, containing natural precursors to female hormones. The hormonal precursors present in shatavari make it a primary menstrual and menopausal regulator. Its tonifying and nourishing effects on the uterus improve reproductive fluids enhancing conception while also

strengthening the muscles of the uterus. Shatavari is moistening and anti-inflammatory.

Slippery elm bark *Ulmus rubra*
The inner bark is full of mucilage which soothes the body's inflamed and irritated mucous membranes and encourages new cellular growth in damaged tissues. Slippery elm is also an anti-inflammatory and antimicrobial, which effectively eliminates toxins through its bulk laxative actions.

Spirulina *Arthrospira platensis*
A microscopic cyanobacteria which is a concentrated source of protein, iron and B Vitamins, spirulina enhances endurance and energy. It is particularly effective where there has been cell damage caused by long-term chronic health conditions.

St John's wort flowering top
Hypericum perforatum Rather erroneously known as a herb that's only good for depression, St John's wort helps to clear stagnant feelings so that you can feel the present instead of the pain of the past or worry of the future. It's a remarkable wound healer that helps us overcome trauma, especially nerve pain. Because highly concentrated extracts can affect the metabolism of some drugs, seek the advice of a herbalist or doctor before using it with medication.

Star anise *Illicium verum* Aromatic,
digestive and calming to inner tension, star anise has a wonderful flavour reminiscent of fennel with bells on.

Thyme leaf *Thymus vulgaris*
High in a volatile oil called thymol that has a *carminative* effect on the digestive system. The oil is also highly antiseptic

and is effective in treating infections both internally and externally. However, it is most famous for strengthening the lungs, helping to clear mucus and reduce wheezing.

Triphala An age-old Ayurvedic remedy
combining amla, bibhitaki and haritaki fruits. It is revered as a decongestant for the digestive system and for cleansing the blood, extending the quality and quantity of life.

Tulsi leaf *Ocimum tenuiflorum*
Light, ascendant and awakening, tulsi leaf (also known as holy basil) creates a sacred space within and without, making it useful for lifting the cloud of minor depression. It's also good for throwing off a chill and is often used on its own as a folk remedy when you feel the early signs of a cold. It's become very popular as a powerful *adaptogen* that helps you adapt to stress and protect your immune system.

Turmeric root *Curcuma longa*
A super-spice par excellence. High in flavonoids and with over 6,000 clinical studies attesting to its ability to protect and nourish the body, it's known to prevent ageing, improve circulation, reduce inflammation, heal wounds and protect the liver and bowels. This golden yellow root is full of the potent flavonoid curcumin and other yellow pigments that act as cellular protectives and systemic rejuvenatives. It has been traditionally used in Ayurveda for over 2,000 years to nourish the joints, digestion, liver, heart, brain and skin. It is pungent, bitter and astringent, and is slightly heating and drying. It has gained the reputation of one of nature's most potent remedies for many of today's health challenges.

Uva ursi leaf *Arctostaphylos uva-ursi*
A famous urinary antiseptic, specific for cystitis or urinary infections. It has a characteristic spicy-sweet smell.

Valerian root *Valeriana officinalis*
Primarily a sedative to help the nervous system alleviate anxiety and chronic insomnia, valerian also relieves muscular tension and is an effective antispasmodic.

Vanilla pod *Vanilla planifolia*
Rich, sweet and aromatic, vanilla is a calming aphrodisiac.

Wheatgrass juice *Triticum aestivum*
This is packed full of chlorophyll, which has a specific ability to rebuild red blood cells. It contains a number of bioactive enzymes which act as catalysts to a wide range of metabolic functions and support energy production and immunity. Wheatgrass also contains a potent antioxidant called superoxide dismutase, which protects against free radicals.

Yarrow top *Achillea millefolium*
Full of contradiction, yarrow will increase circulation but also stop bleeding and leakage. It will get a sluggish period going or slow a menstrual period that is flowing too quickly. It helps induce a sweat when there is fever and stop diarrhoea when there is an upset tummy.

Yellow dock root *Rumex crispus*
A bittersweet tonic for the liver that acts as an *alterative* healer to cleanse the organs that work to eliminate waste in the body: liver, bowel and kidneys. It's a gentle laxative helping to stimulate the bowel by encouraging the liver to secrete bile. It is used to cleanse the blood and when the blood is weakened by a torpid liver.

Where do herbs come from?

With much of the world depending on herbs as their primary source of health support, you can just imagine the huge volumes we harvest. Millions of tonnes each year. Around 80 per cent of all herbal species come from the wild, and around 30 per cent of the volume of herbs we harvest are from the wild (the remaining 70 per cent are cultivated). Rather worryingly, around 10,000 of the 50,000 medicinal herbs we use are thought to be threatened in their natural habitats due to overharvesting and habitat loss. And as we all reawaken to the power of plants, the need for greater awareness about where our herbs come from and how they are grown should move to top of the agenda. In fact, it's up to us to do something about it.

Unsustainable extraction is usually driven by demand – often by companies or consumers who are unaware that they are buying or using threatened species. This means that we can all play an important role in plant conservation, simply by choosing sustainably sourced products in the shops. We have the choice and that gives us the power. That coin in your hand is a vote for how you want our world to be.

For example, most licorice grows in the wild and is subject to overharvesting – do you want to buy any old licorice or do you want to know exactly where it comes from and how sustainably it has been harvested? Do you want pesticide-covered peppermint or naturally grown organic peppermint? Unfortunately, it's a sorry affair and many species have been exploited for far too long.

Going back to licorice (*Glycyrrhiza glabra* and *uralensis*), that grows all over the world – it even used to be grown in the UK in Pontefract, West Yorkshire. Historically a large portion of the global supply has come from China and Turkey. Its increased popularity and lack of controls on harvesting mean that China and Turkey are now suffering from declining availability and even a shortage of wild licorice. Similarly echinacea, goldenseal and American ginseng have all become endangered in the wild in America due to overharvesting brought on by consumer demand.

It's easy to know if your herbs are sustainably sourced if they carry certain certification logos identifying that there have been appropriate checks on their harvesting. The Soil Association in the UK is unique among organic certification agencies in that they require verification that all herbs harvested from the wild are from a sustainable source. Another logo is the FairWild certification scheme that ensures appropriate monitoring, resource assessments and management of the plants and people involved in collection. These are the gold standards of herb conservation and sustainable herb growing today.

But what about herbs that are cultivated? Are they all 'good' because they are 'natural'?

Growing organic herbs

I am a committed supporter of the principles and benefits of organic farming. Organic means much more than just the absence of agrochemicals – it is a method of growing crops ensuring that we give back as much as we take, of creating cycles of benefit at each stage of the journey from field to shelf and of treading lightly on our planet. It's also the fairest system of agriculture in the world as it benefits the soil, water, plants, animals and humans equally. It's a system of farming that means we take responsibility for our impact on the planet now and don't leave a mess for our children to clean up.

You will probably be amazed to hear that most herbs available today are grown with pesticides, herbicides and synthetic fertilisers. This is a completely unnecessary and wasteful practice that not only damages the environment but also reduces the potency of the herbs. It's been shown in multiple studies that organic crops generate higher levels of protective phytochemical antioxidant compounds than conventional crops. Because the plants in an organic system are exposed to the 'elements' they have to fend for themselves, and this makes them develop stronger defences. So organic is better for the planet, better for the plants and better for you. Organic is about looking after the whole. And these organic principles looking at the sustainability of life are at the heart of Ayurveda, India's traditional healthcare system. They are also the principles that inspire Pukka's purpose, which is to help people connect to the power of plants.

Herb suppliers

UK

Baldwins
www.baldwins.co.uk

Indigo Herbals
www.indigo-herbs.co.uk

Neal's Yard Remedies
www.nealsyardremedies.com

Organic Herb Trading Company
www.organicherbtrading.com
(for 500g or more)

Pukka Herbs
www.pukkaherbs.com
(for specialist Ayurvedic herbs in
quantaties of 500g or more)

USA

Banyan Botanicals
www.banyanbotanicals.com
(specialist Ayurvedic herbs)

Herbalist and Alchemist
www.herbalist-alchemist.com

Mountain Rose
www.mountainroseherbs.com

Practitioners & herbal organisations

If you are interested in exploring how herbs can help you heal, I strongly recommend that you work with a qualified professional for treatment. For help in finding one, explore these resources:

UK

Association of Master Herbalists
www.associationofmaster
herbalists.co.uk

Ayurvedic Practitioners Association
Tel: 0044 (0)1273 500 492
www.apa.uk.com

National Institute of Medical Herbalists
Tel: 0044 (0)1392 426 022
www.nimh.org.uk

Register of Chinese Herbal Medicine
Tel: 0044 (0)1603 623 994
www.rchm.co.uk

Unified Register of Herbal Practitioners
Tel: 0044 (0)1872 222 699
www.urhp.org

USA

American Herbalists Guild
www.americanherbalistsguild.com

National Ayurvedic Medical Association
www.ayurveda-nama.org

Index

A

aches 2, 135, 154, *see also* pain
acid in stomach 29, 59, 60, 95, 127, 216, *see also* digestive system
acids, fatty 193–4, 225–6
acne 28, 36, 183
adaptogens 27, 69, 127, 199, 226, 230
ADHD (attention deficit hyperactivity disorder) 28
adrenaline 39
adrenals 55, 83, 89, 127, 162, 222, 226
ailments 28, 39
alcohol 42, 187, 200, 216
alcohol withdrawal 28
allergies 28, 225, 228
allopathic medicine 27
almond 29, *70, 73, 193,* 222
aloe vera 13, 16, 27, *60, 196,* 216, 222
alteratives 27, 36, 46, 74, 183, 218, 223, 230
Alzheimer's 28
amla 7, 27, *64, 151, 188, 199,* 222, 230
amphoterics 27
andrographis 16, *35,* 219
angelica *77–8,* 222
angostura 42
aniseed *20,* 27, *39, 138–43,* 222
anti–dyspeptic remedies 127
anti–hepatotoxic remedies 127
anti–inflammatory remedies 39, 95, 127, 154, 175, 193, 211, 216, 219, 222, 225–8, 230
anti–ulcer remedies 64, 95, 127, 154, 227
antibacterial remedies 127, 137, 157, 224–5, 227–8
antibiotic properties 11, 147
antidepressant remedies 224, *see also* depression
antiemetic remedies 52, *see also* nausea
antifungal remedies 224–5, 228
antimicrobials 15, 27, 45, 95, 135, 147, 219, 223, 225, 230
antioxidants 12, 52, 64, 99, 100, 107, 108, 115, 123, 124, 140, 151, 199, 216,

222–6, 228–30, 231
antispasmodic remedies 59, 95, 222, 224, 230
antiviral remedies 127, 140, 225, 227
anxiety 16, 93, 95, 104, 115, 116, 170, 176, 212, 218, 222, 227–30 *see also* stress
aperients 27, *see also* laxatives
aphrodisiac 27, 70, 73, 83, 162, 219, 222, 227, 230
Aphrodite's Aphrodisiac 162
appetite 50, 217, 219
arthritis 16, 28, 74, 154, 228
artichoke 35
ashwagandha 12, 16, 27, 69, *73, 77–8, 154, 162, 200,* 222
asthma 28
astragalus *77–8, 200,* 222
astringent remedies 45, 60, 63, 64, 74, 89, 107, 108, 116, 119, 123, 124, 154, 165, 166, 213, 214, 215, 219–20, 222, 226, 228–30
attention deficit hyperactivity disorder (ADHD) 28
Ayurveda 7, 9, 13, 19, 27, 32, 39, 50, 52, 59, 64, 68, 70, 77, 93, 99, 100, 130, 134, 138, 140, 151, 166, 169, 188, 191, 211–20, 229, 231
    constitutions 25, 27, 39, 59, 80, 169, 211, *see also* vata, pitta, kapha, doshas
    physician, Charaka 7, 70, 134
    tastes 213–20
    temperature 213, 214

B

back pain 175, 225
bacteria 11, 15, 27, 127, 135, 137, 148, 157, 219, 224–5, 227–8, 230
basil, holy (tulsi) 16, *99, 138,* 187, 226, 230
bee balm, *see* lemon balm
beetroot 15, *77–8,* 215, 222
bhringraj *153,* 222
bibhitaki *64,* 222, 230

bilberry *151, 199,* 223
bile 27, 33, 35, 39, 40, 216, 218, 222, 227, 230
    aids 35, 39, 40, 216, 218, 222, 227, 230
black tea *23, 84,* 226
bladder, *see also* urinary system
    aids 29, 45, 214, 224
bleeding gums 28
bleeding 74, 165, 217, 220, 229, 230
Bliss Of The Gods 124
bloating 32, 39, 59, 64, 95, 104, 165, 223
blood 77, 78, *see also* blood poisoning; blood pressure; blood sugar
    aids 15, 52, 73, 74, 84, 123, 148, 154, 165, 166, 175, 193, 196, 199, 215, 218, 222–24, 226–7, 229
    ailments 15, 27, 170, 194, 199, 216, 217, 218, 219, 225
    cleansing 36, 39, 46, 64, 140, 219, 228, 222–3, 230
blood poisoning 28, 140
blood pressure 27, 28, 46, 123, 128, 193, 212, 217, 226–8
blood sugar regulation 28, 84, 108, 224
boils 28
Boswellia *154,* 218, 223
bowels 33, 50
    aids 27, 36, 40, 219, 220, 227, 229, 230
    ailments 64, *see also* irritable bowel syndrome
brain 15, 193, 212
    aids 15, 19, 70, 99, 100, 107, 116, 119, 124, 170, 215, 222, 226, 229, 230
Brave Heart 123
breastfeeding 27, 28, 74, 169, 170, 227, 229
Breathe 138
breathing 69, 93, 138, 212
    aids 137, 138, 157, 227
    ailments 32, 33, 138, 157, 216
bronchitis 28, 216, *see also* breathing
bruises 15
buchu *45,* 223
burdock 27, *36, 46, 183,* 215, 223

C

cacao 27, *83, 124, 162,* 224
Cacao Orange Rejuvenator 83
caffeine 12, 89, 107, 119
calcium 12, 74, 78, 104, 183, 222, 224, 229
candida 28
cannabis, *see* hemp
carbon 12
cardamom *20, 39, 70–3, 84, 86, 99, 104, 193,* 218, 223
cardiovascular health 12, 15, 16, 226, 228, *see also* heart
carminatives 27, 35, 39, 52, 56, 115, 217, 222–25, 228, 230, *see also* digestive system
cataracts 151
catarrh 28, 220
catnip 180, 223
celery 196
celery seed *20,* 27, *39, 154,* 217, 223
CFS (chronic fatigue syndrome) 28
chamomile 13, 16, 20, *23, 60, 95, 96, 100–04, 165, 170, 176, 179–80,* 216, 219, 223
Charaka 7, 70, 134
chasteberry 27, 165
chest
    aids 123, 137, 157, 201, 227–8
    ailments 13, 28, 52, 89, 135, 138, 143, 157, 180, 212, 216, 227–8
chicory 83, 224
children 25, 95, 115, 160–1, 169, 176, 179, 180, 223, 231
Chinese medicine 7
chlorella 16, 217, 224
chlorophyll 36, 107, 196, 230
chocolate *see* cacao
cholagogue 35 *see also* bile
cholesterol 27, 63, 194, 218, 223, 225–6
chronic fatigue syndrome (CFS) 28
chrysanthemum *151,* 224
cinnamon 13, 20, *23,* 25, 50, *63, 86–9, 123–4, 137, 144, 162, 200,* 214, 216, 218, 220, 224

circulation 13, 27, 42, 52, 55, 73, 89, 123, 130, 137, 143, 147–51, 154, 162, 165, 180, 188, 199, 200, 214, 222–6, 229–30
Clean Greens 196
cleansing herbs 9, 32–47, 64, 74, 100, 130, 140, 147, 151, 183, 196, 217, 219, 222–5, 230
cloves 124, 137, 144
cocoa bean *see* cacao
colds 28, 32, 130, 135, 140, 148, 157, 201, 225, 230
communication 27, 212
compounds 11, 12, 23, 33, 100, 107, 119, 124, 137, 187, 199, 218, 224, 226, 231, *see also* antioxidants; caffeine; essential oils; steroids
congestion 32, 35, 46, 74, 138, 140, 144, 188, 212, 216, 218, 222–23, 225–27
constipation 27, 28, 64, 212, 219, 228
Cool Chamomile 95
Cool Lady 170–3
Cool Waters 45
coriander *45, 59, 169, 188–91, 196,* 224
corn silk 27, *45,* 214–15, 224
cough 16, 28, 33, 35, 55, 127, 133, 135, 138, 144, 157, 180, 215, 224
cramp bark (guelder rose) 16, *175,* 224
cranberry *45,* 217, 224
Culpeper, Nicholas 7
cumin 188, *191,* 224, 230
A Cup Of Love 96
cuts 15
cyanobacteria 11, 230
cystitis 28, 36, *45,* 74, 215, 230

D

damiana *162,* 224
dandelion 15, 16, 19, *20,* 35–40, *45,* 27, 83, *165, 183,* 219, 224–5
dandruff 153
decongestant remedies 56, 223, 230
dehydration *45,* 217
demulcents 27, 40, 60, 80, 127, 215, 217, 224, 226–8

depression 28, 32, 73, 123, 212, 224, 228–30, *see also* anxiety; stress
detoxing 20, 32–47, 64, 74, 78, 154, 157, 196, 217–18, 219, 222–4, 229
diabetes 27, 84, 108, 212, 216
diaphoretics 27, 56, 148, 223
diarrhoea 32, 188, 214, 220, 226, 228, 230
digestive system 12, 15, 20, 27, 32–42, 50–64, 73, 80, 104, 135, 212, 214, 216–20, 222–5, 227–30
    aids 9, 15, 19, 27, 35, 39, 40, 42, 50–64, 70, 73, 80–9, 95, 104, 107, 115, 120, 127, 130, 135, 138, 147, 157, 165, 166,188–96, 212, 214, 216–17, 218-19, 220, 222–5, 227–30
    ailments 12, 32, 35, 36, 39, 40, 56, 59, 60, 80, 95, 104, 120, 127, 166, 173, 175, 179, 180, 199, 214, 217, 222–5, 227–30
Digestive Detox With A Twist 20, 39
Digestive Lassi 191
diuretics 19, 27, 35, 36, 45, 46, 154, 215, 216, 219, 223–4, 226
dizziness 217, 218, 219
dosages 24, 25, 217
doshas 169, 199, 211, 215, 220, 225–6, 229
drugs 12, 28, 33, 113, 144, 230
dryness 16, 104, 127, 137, 162, 173, 214, 216, 218, 220, 226
dysmenorrhoea 28

E

Eagle Eyes 151
echinacea 27, *140–3,* 216, 217, 225, 231
eczema 28, 74, 211
elderberry 13, 27, *140–3, 144, 151, 180, 199, 201,* 217, 225
Elderberry And Echinacea Winter Warmer 140–3
Elderberry Elixir 144
elderflower 15, 27, *140, 147–8, 180,* 225
elecampane 16, 27
electrolyte balance 19, 46, 128
emmenagogues 27, 227

endometriosis 28
essential oils 9, 12, 19, 40, 56, 59, 63, 73,
    83, 95, 99, 100, 115, 120, 124, 130,
    137, 140–3, 148, 151, 157, 169, 173, 179,
    191, 218
expectorants 27, 127, 143, 144, 216, 222,
    227
eyes 68, 151, 193, 217
    aids 151, 196, 223–4, 226
    ailments 28, 95, 151, 224

F
fatigue 28, 32, 33, 35, 127, 165
fatty acids 15, 183, 193–4, 225–6
fennel 27, 50, *20, 35–40, 46, 59, 104, 151,
    166–75, 179, 193*, 216, 225
fertility 12, 27, 28, 160, 162, 169, 188, 212,
    222, *see also* infertility
fertiliser 23, 231
fevers 27, 140, 148, 180, 216, 217, 223,
    225, 230
fieldmint 56
Fire Extinguisher 60
flatulence 27, 28, 52, 64, 104, 179, 212,
    217, 220
flax seed 27, 194
flushes, hot 27, 170, 212
flu 13, 28, 144, 148, 225
Forgive Me For I Have Sinned 42
frankincense 154, 218
Fruits Of The Forest 201
Full Moon Celebrations 166
fungi 27, 135

G
galactagogues 27, 169, 227
galangal *55*, 225
Galen 7
gall–bladder 27, 35, 214
garlic 15, 214, 218
gastritis 95
ghee *188*, 225
ginger 15, 20, *23*, 27, *42, 55*, 63, *84–9, 104,
    124, 137–48, 154, 175, 180, 188–91, 196,*
200, 205, 214, 215, 218, 225–6
The Ginger Princess 205
Ginger The Great 52
gingerols 52, 225
ginkgo 19
ginseng 13, 16, 19, 27, 69, *83, 200,*
    226, 231
goji berry *151,* 226
gokshura *46,* 226
Golden Milk Of Bliss 73
The Golden Ginger Triangle 55
golden seal 231
goldenrod 46
A Good Move 40
gotu kola 15, 226
gout 28, 39, 154
Greek medicine 7
Green Matcha Zen 107
green tea 23, *63, 89, 107, 108, 119,
    202,* 226
guelder rose 16, *see also* cramp bark
gynaecological 16, *see also* women's
    health

H
haemorrhoids 28, 64
hair 28, 153, 216, 217, 222, 227
halitosis 28
haritaki 27, *64,* 220, 226, 230
hawthorn 15, *123, 201,* 215, 226
hayfever 28, 225
head 56, 103, 116, 153, 170, 200, 214
    ailments 33, 42, 83, 99, 115, 138, 140,
        157, 224, 227–8
heart 123, 215, 218
    aids 15, 16, 96, 116, 119, 123, 214, 215,
        226, 228
    ailments 15, 16, 27, 29, 96, 123, 124,
        170, 199, 212, 218, 220
heartburn 27, 29, 60, 211, 212,
    see also digestive system
Heavenly Empress Vitality Tonic 77–8
Help Me Glow 36
hemp *193–4, 199,* 226

hepatics 27
herbalism
    energetic 11, 13
    natural 11–12
    phytochemical 11, 12
hibiscus 59, 165
Hippocrates 7
hives 29
holistic health 211*see also* Ayurveda
honey *42, 56, 70, 73, 83, 116, 124, 137–8,
    147, 154, 162, 176–83,* 187, *193, 199, 201,*
    205, 216, 227
hormones 27, 95, 123, 154, 162, 165, 169,
    170, 183, 193, 212, 213, 226, 229
horsemint 56
horseradish 16
horsetail *153,* 226
Huang Di 7
hydrogen 12
hyperactivity 115

I
IBS (irritable bowel syndrome) 29, 93
I Love My Liver 35
Illustriously Lustrous Locks 153
immune system 12, 28, 32, 69, 144
    aids 55, 78, 134–5, 140, 147, 148, 154,
        180, 194, 196, 199, 201, 215, 222–3,
        225, 227, 229–30
Incredible Immunity 148
indigestion 60, 64, 95, 211, 212, 217, 222,
    224, *see also* digestive system
infection 32, 45, 130, 135, 140, 147, 148,
    180, 199, 212, 215, 216, 219, 222–6, 230
infertility 27, 212, *see also* fertility
inflammation 27, 32, 35, 52, 64, 95, 127,
    130, 135, 154, 165, 175, 193, 194, 199,
    212, 214, 217, 219, 220, 222, 225–30
insomnia 27, 29, 73, 93, 170, 212, 222,
    227–8, 230
iron 74, 77–8, 183, 196, 222
irritability 27, 176
irritable bowel syndrome (IBS) 29, 93
itchiness 32, 36, 153, 217, 219

J

jasmine 216, 226
Jasmine Green Tea 119
Joint Protector 154
joints 193, 223, 230
 ailments 16, 39, 52, 74, 154

K

kapha 25, 27, 89, 127, 130, 188, 211, 212,
 214–20, 225
kidneys 27, 29, 33, 46
 aids 36, 39, 46, 80, 214, 223–4, 226, 230
 ailments 29, 32, 39, 218, 226

L

lavender *96–103, 116,* 227
laxatives 27, 40, 64, 166, 215, 217, 219,
 226, 228, 230
legs *see* RLS
Lemon And Ginger With Manuka Honey
 147
lemon balm (melissa) 13, 20, *23, 115–16,*
 120, 176, 228
Lemon Heaven 120
lemon juice 20, 29, 36, 39, 120, 147, 196,
 205, 216, 227
lemongrass *120, 138, 169,* 218, 227
Let There Be Joy 116
Li Shizhen 7
licorice 16, 20, *23, 27, 35–40, 55, 59–60,*
 80–3, 86–89, 96, 100–04, 127–8, 137,
 140–3, 154, 162–5, 170, 173, 183, 202,
 215, 227, 231
Light On Tulsi 130
lime juice 204
limeflower 27, *96, 103, 116, 123, 176,* 227
Linnaeus 16
linseed *193,* 227
lion's tooth *see* dandelion
Little One's Calm Cup 176
Little One's Cold Tea 180
Little One's Tummy Tea 179
liver 27, 29, 33, 36, 35, 214
 aids 27, 35–42, 78, 107, 120, 157, 165,

 194, 199, 216, 219, 222, 225, 229, 230
 ailments 15, 29, 32
lungs 33
 aids 20, 27, 55, 137–44, 180, 230
 ailments 29, 39, 56, 104, 127, 143, 180,
 215, 216, 219, 223, 227

M

maca 162, 227
magnesium 12, 74, 124, 196
Maharaja's Majestic Chai 84
Majestic Mint 56
Manuka honey *137, 147,* 216, 227
marigold 27, *96, 151,* 227
marshmallow 27, *40, 45–6, 60, 104, 137,*
 214, 216
meadowsweet 60, 154
medicine, *see also* Ayurveda
 allopathic 27
 Chinese 7, 19, 35
 Greek 7
 western herbal 19, 27
melissa, *see* lemon balm
Melissa's Magic 115
memory 68, 99, *see also* brain; aids
 aids 15, 99, 170, 229
menopause 29, 77, 160, 170, 228,
 see also flushes, hot
menstrual cramps 16, 96, 224, 227–9
menstruation
 aids 16, 27, 29, 124, 165
 ailments 165, 173, 230
mental alertness 42, 99, 162, 227,
 see also brain
metabolic waste 27, 32–3, 39
metabolism 55, 63, 108, 143, 193, 196,
 212, 214, 218, 223–5, 230
 aids 27, 42, 52, 55, 63, 108, 143, 165,
 193, 196, 212, 223–5, 230
metabolites 12
migraine 29
minerals 19, 23, 45, 46, 74, 77–8, 107,
 124, 153, 183, 193, 196, 199, 217, 222,
 225, 227–8

mint *16, 56, 130, 196, 202, 204,* 229,
 see also catnip; peppermint
Mint Digestif 59
molasses 77–8, 153
Monthly Liberation 175
Moon Balance 165
morphine 12
motherwort 16, *123, 165,* 228
Mother's Milk 169
mouth 213, 216, 219
mouth ulcers 29
movement 27, 212
mucilage 27, 40, 45, 60, 137, 230, 165, 224
mucus 13, 15, 27, 39, 55, 84, 138–47, 180,
 188, 212, 215–6, 219, 220, 223, 225,
 227, 230
muscle strain/ache 29, 32, 52, 56, 104,
 175, 219
muscles skeletal 15, 214, 215
 aids 27, 46, 214, 215, 226, 228, 230
myalgic encephalomyelitis (ME) 29
myrrh 11

N

Natural Balance 63
nausea 15, 32, 33, 52, 175, 179, 226
neem 16, *35,* 219, 228
nervines 27, 165, 224
nervous system 12, 170, 193, 212, 215, 217,
 219, 222
 aids 20, 27, 55, 70, 73, 80, 83, 93, 95,
 100, 103, 104, 127, 162, 175, 183,
 224, 227–30
nettle 20, 27, *36,* 74–8, *153, 166, 183,* 228
nitrogen 12
Nourishing Almond Saffron Elixir 70
Nourishing Nettle Tea 74
nutmeg *73,* 228
nutrients 15, 50, 52, 59, 77, 78, 104, 140, 179,
 191, 193, 196, 214, 220, 222, 225, 229

O

oat straw flowering tops 27, *103, 104,*
 183, 228

obesity 29, 63, 216

olive leaf 100

oolong 23, 108, 226

orange recipes 40, 63, 83, 124, 140–3, 200

organic herbs 8, 19, 23, 50, 60, 83, 137, 158, 188, 231

osteoporosis 29

osteroarthritis see arthritis

P

pain 45, 52, 59–60, 64, 95, 96, 124, 135, 154, 165, 175, 212, 220, 222, 224–5, 227, 229

parasitic infections 219, 226

passion flower 27, 170, 228

pathogens 15

PCOS (poly cystic ovarian syndrome) 29

Peace Tea 100

pepper, black 63, 196, 214, 218, 223

peppermint 12, 27, 36, 42, 56–9, 80, 138, 140, 148, 166, 179–83, 231

Peppermint And Licorice 80

periods 27, 29, 33, 52, 74, 95, 160, 165, 175, 212, 230

pesticides 19, 23, 33, 231

phlegm 29, 137, 138, 143, 157, 214

phosphorus 12, 74

physicians, historic 7

phytochemicals 11, 12, 15, 193, 231

phytonutrients 196, 199

piles 29

pitta 27, 59, 95, 127, 188, 211, 212, 214, 215, 216, 217, 218–20, 222

plant

   colour 15, 16, 19, 229

   conservation 231

   signatures 15–16

plantain 45

PMS (premenstrual syndrome) 29, 165

poisons 33, 140, 219, 225

pollen 95, 162, 225

pollen, flower 95, 162, 225

poly cystic ovarian syndrome (PCOS) 29

polyphenols 107, 108, 219, 226

pomegranate 123, 199, 207, 217, 228

potassium 19, 45, 74

prana 13, 77, 99, 138, 220, 228

pregnancy 12, 29, 74, 128, 166

premenstrual syndrome (PMS) 29, 165

prostate 29, 226

psoriasis 29, 74

psyllium 64, 228

Pukka teas 8, 196, 199, 202, 204, 207, 213, 217–19, 220

Pukkalini 207

Pure Clarity 99

Q

qi 13, 222

R

rashes 27, 29, 212, 222

raspberry 166, 201, 220, 228

red clover 36, 170, 228

rejuvenation 7, 13, 64, 68–89, 99, 100, 127, 128, 140, 151, 162, 166, 169, 199, 200, 216, 222, 225–6, 230

remedies

   adaptogen 27, 69, 127, 199, 226, 230

   alterative 27, 36, 46, 74, 183, 218, 223, 230

   amphoteric 27

   antibiotic 11, 147

   anti–dyspeptic 127

   anti–hepatotoxic 127

   anti–inflammatory 39, 95, 127, 154, 175, 193, 211, 216, 219, 222, 225–230

   anti–ulcer 64, 95, 127, 154, 227

   antibacterial 127, 137, 157, 224–5, 227–8

   antidepressant 224, see also depression

   antiemetic 52, see also nausea

   antifungal 224–5, 228

   antimicrobial 15, 27, 45, 95, 135, 147, 219, 223, 225, 230

   antioxidant 12, 52, 64, 99, 100, 107, 108, 115, 123, 124, 140, 144, 151, 199,

216, 222–6, 228–9, 231

   antispasmodic 59, 95, 222, 224, 230

   antiviral 127, 140, 225, 227

   aphrodisiac 27, 70, 73, 83, 162, 219, 222, 227, 230

   astringent 45, 60, 63, 64, 74, 89, 107, 108, 116, 119, 123, 124, 154, 165, 166, 213, 214, 215, 219–20, 222, 226, 228–9, 230

   carminative 27, 35, 39, 52, 56, 115, 217, 222–25, 228, 230, see also digestive system

   decongestant 56, 223, 230

   demulcent 27, 40, 60, 80, 127, 215, 217, 224, 226–28

   diaphoretic 27, 56, 148, 223

   diuretic 19, 27, 35, 36, 45, 46, 154, 215, 216, 219, 223–4, 226

   emmenagogue 27, 227

   expectorant 27, 127, 143, 144, 216, 222, 227

   galactagogue 27, 169, 227

   hepatic 27

   laxative 27, 40, 64, 166, 215, 217, 219, 226, 228, 230

   mucilage 27, 40, 45, 60, 137, 230, 165, 224

   nervine 27, 165, 224

reproductive health 29, 33, 70, 78, 104, 160–5, 215, 216, 222, 226

respiratory disorders 12, 15, 27, 144, 201, 223, 225

respiratory system 12, 15, 27, 138, 144, 201, 223, 225

   aids 144, 225, see also breathing

restless leg syndrome (RLS) 29, 95, 223

Rise Like A Star 89

RLS (restless leg syndrome) 29, 95, 223

rose 60, 96, 123, 165, 188, 207, 229

Rose Essence Lassi 188

rose water 116, 124, 188, 207

rosehip 140, 201, 229

rosemary 35, 42, 99, 116, 153, 157, 200, 229

Rosemary And Thyme 157

A Royal Flush 46

S

saffron 27, *70*, *73*, *123*, *193*, 229
sage *170*, 215, 229
salt 196, 213, 215, 217, 220
Sanskrit 16, 50, 80, 213
schisandra berries *35*, 229
seaweed *196*, 217, 229
The Seeds Of life 193–4
semen, reduction of 219
senna 25, 27, *40*, 229
sex 27, 73, 162
shatavari 7, 16, 27, 69, *77–8*, *162–70*, 215, 229, 230
shinrin–yoku 13
shogaols 52, 225–6
signatures, plant 15–16, 63
Sing A Song 137
sinus problems 29, 222
skin 33, 56, 77
    aids 39, 56, 68, 108, 148, 183, 196, 215, 225, 227
    ailments 27, 29, 32, 36, 39, 64, 74, 96, 212, 217, 219, 223, 228
sleep 13, 73, 95, 103, 176, 222, 227–8
slippery elm 27, *60*, *137*, 230
snake bite 140, 225
sodium 128
sodium bicarbonate 45
spasms 27, 52, 59, 80, 95, 104, 165, 166, 175, 179, 222, 224, 229
spearmint recipes 56, 89, 99–100
spirulina 11, 16, 217, 230
St John's Wort 15, *116*, 230
star anise *89*, 216, 218, 230
steroids 12, 39
stomach 53, 214, 229 *see also* digestive system
    ailments 27, 29, 40, 59, 60, 80, 95, 104, 54, 179, 216
stress 27, 29, 32, 33, 39, 69, 83, 93, 95, 104, 222, 226, 228, 230,
        see also anxiety; depression
sugar 78, 86, 128, 144, 215, 216
sugar levels 63, 84, 108, 224

A Supremely Wild Sparkler 202
Sushruta 7
sweat 27, 56, 140, 147, 148, 170, 214, 215, 218, 220, 225, 229–30
Sweet Dreams 103
Sweet Herb Chai 86
Sweet Licorice 127–8

T

Take It Easy 104
taste 16, 213–20
teenagers 183
Three Mint Matcha Mojito 204
throat, sore 29, 52, 135, 137, 144, 216, 225, 227
thyme 20, 27, *138*, *157*, 230
thyroid 211, 115, 196
tongue 213, 215, 216, 217, 219
    ailments 32, 64
tonsillitis 29, *see also* throat, sore
Too Cool For School 183
trauma 96, 226, 230
travel sickness 29
triphala tea *63*, *64*, *199*, 199, 217, 220, 230
Triphala Tea 64
tulsi 13, 16, 27, *99*, *130*, *138*, *148*, 218, 230
tummy *see also* stomach; digestive system
    ailments 12, 40, 60, 95, 175, 179, 230
turmeric 15, 23, 27, *35–6*, *42*, *55*, *63*, *73*, *147*, *151*, *154*, *175*, *196*, 230

U

ulcers 64, 95, 127, 154, 217, 227
uric acid 39
urinary system 39, 216, 223, 225–6, 227
    aids 27, 39, 45, 215, 216, 223–5, 227, 230
    ailments 29, 39, 45, 74, 104, 180, 215, 224, 226, 230
uterus
    aids 95, 165, 166, 175, 224, 228, 230
    ailments 95, 175
uva ursi *45*, 230

V

valerian *103*, *175*, 230
vanilla *86*, *124*, *162*, *165*, 216, 230
vata 25, 27, 95, 104, 127, 130, 188, 211–12, 214–20, 222, 228
verbena *23*, *120*, 227
viruses 13, 15, 27, 135, 144, 147, 148, 201, 225
vis medicatrix naturae 13
Vitalise Berry Boost 199
vitamins 78, 140, 144, 147, 151, 166, 183, 193, 196, 199, 201, 211, 216, 217, 222, 225, 227–30

W

walnuts 15 *193*, *194*
water retention 29, 32, 188, 217
weight 25, 27, 29, 63, 108, 194, 196, 212, 216, 219
western herbal medicine 19, 27
wetness 16
wheatgrass *196*, 230
willow 15, 16
wind *see* flatulence
Winter Tonic Elixir 200
Winter Warmer, Elderberry And Echinacea 140–3
women's health 16, 29, 33, 70, 77–8, 95, 124, 160–75, 193–4, 220, 228
wounds 11, 12, 116, 214, 216, 219, 220, 226, 230

Y

yarrow 15, 27, *148*, 230
yellow dock root 27, *40*, *77–8*, 230

Index

Thank yous

There is a traditional Ayurvedic tale that every single plant in the world has special healing benefits – all you have to do is learn about their character. I can't disagree with this as I have certainly found a deep sense of wonder in the wisdom of plants. That we are connected with nature in so many ways and on such a profound level is testament to the oneness of life. With this in mind I am offering this book to all the healing plants of the world.

I would also like to offer this book to you, the Pukka tea drinker. May you find the right herbs to help you flourish.

And finally a big thank you to all the people who have made it possible for me to be a vessel for sharing the herbal wisdom of our ancestors: Susie and Emerson for their enduring sense of humour and enlightening wisdom; to everyone at Pukka Herbs for their remarkable expertise, enthusiasm and vision; to Tim for his commitment to the cause; to Fox for his creative insights; and to Suresh from Sprung Sultan for his watchful guidance. Also to Zena my commissioning editor from Frances Lincoln and her fantastic team of designers, photographers and proofreaders for helping pull it all together.

Sebastian Pole co-founded Pukka Herbs in 2001. He is a global spokesperson for Ayurveda, organic farming and herbal remedies. He is a trained practitioner in Ayurveda, Traditional Chinese Medicine and Western Herbalism, as well as a qualified yoga teacher and therapist.

He is the author of *A Pukka Life* and *Ayurvedic Medicine*.

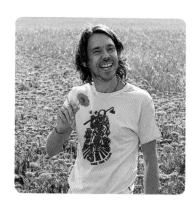

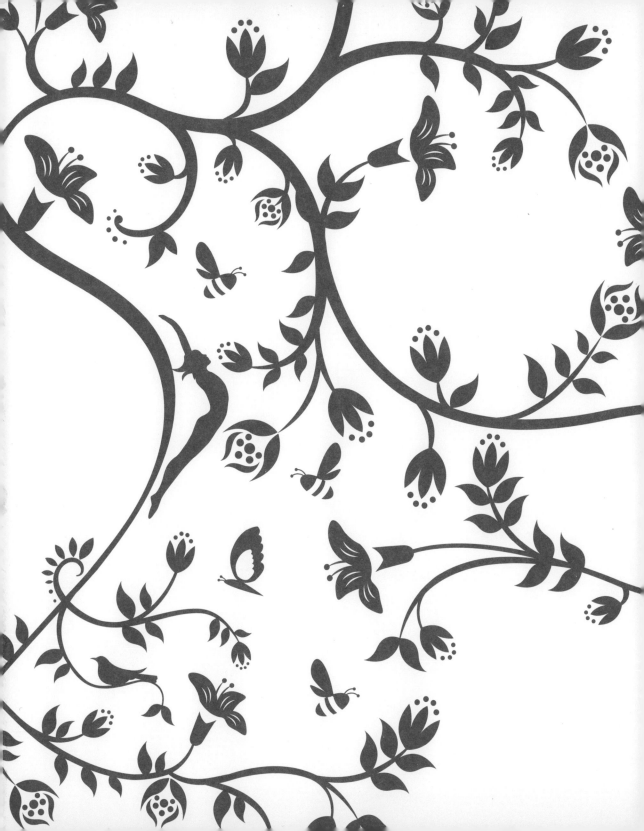

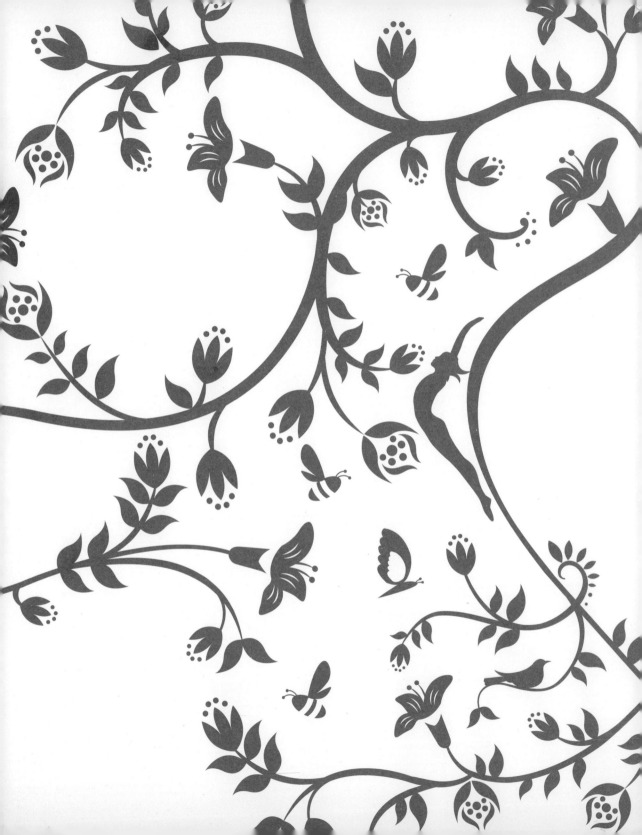